It's Definitely Breast Cancer

First-hand experience of
what actually works and
the journey getting there

Sharon Ratchford

Copyright 2017

It's Definitely Breast Cancer
by Sharon Ratchford

FIRST EDITION

Printed in the United States of America

ISBN 9781944265007

FORESIGHT BOOK PUBLISHING
ForesightPublishingNow.com

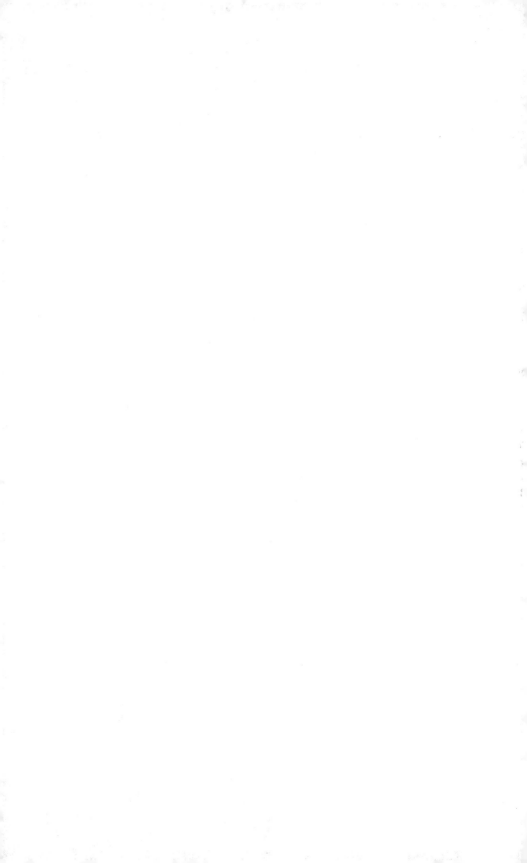

TABLE OF CONTENTS

DISCLAIMER:

I am not an oncology professional. Everything within the pages of this book is based on my personal experience with breast cancer and the research that followed. This book should be considered as support/supplemental material and should not be substituted for the advice of a medical professional. The reader should regularly consult a physician in matters relating to his/her health and particularly with respect to any symptoms that may require diagnosis or medical attention. References are provided for informational purposes only and do not constitute endorsement of any websites or other sources. Readers should be aware that the websites listed in this book are subject to change since the date of publication.

DEDICATION

My God — For His promise to never leave nor forsake me and for reasons far too numerous to list. With You all things are possible.

Alana — My precious daughter, you are my constant source of joy. Your faith never wavered through all the tears, laughter, and the many emotions we went through together; you never doubted mommy would get better. Words cannot express how much I love you. You are truly a gift from God.

Dan — My husband and best friend. You make me laugh, you take care of me, and you helped me through the darkest days of my life. You gave unlimited devotion and loved me through everything (even baldness). I cherish our relationship and love you with all my heart.

Mom — You took care of me and never left my side when I needed you the most. I cannot imagine how often you worried but you stayed strong through every surgery, complication, and set back. I strive to be an amazing mom just like you.

Daddy — You stayed with me from the first day we learned I had cancer. Your strength, encouragement, and never failing love got me through more than I knew possible. I can never thank you enough for all you've done for me but always know I love you and I am so proud to be your daughter.

Aunt Linda — You have the greatest servant's heart, you're always helping someone. But whatever was happening in your world stopped the day I was diagnosed. You were with me every step of the way. Your faith in my healing never faltered. I love you so very much.

Sandra — *my sister* — You and the girls mean more to me than I can express. You knew my favorites and always made certain I had plenty of potato soup. I am forever grateful for all you did. You also graciously fought your own battle and know firsthand God is so very good.

Dolores — "The prayer of the righteous person is powerful and effective" (James 5:16 NIV). When the Bible refers to the righteous I envision you. You consistently prayed for me, cared for us, and did more than I could possibly write. God truly blessed me the day I joined your family.

My extended sisters — You took care of us and were always ready to help in any way. Your love and friendship mean the world to me. "In-law" could never describe our relationship. I thank God for giving me such wonderful sisters, nieces, and nephews. I cherish you with all my heart.

My goddaughter — Our families are one. We love, support, and carry each other through anything life brings our way. I am so very proud to be your godmother.

Our squad — "Friend" does not describe our relationship. You know who you are. Mere words cannot express my gratitude for all you did for us and how much you mean to me. We share life experiences, we talk about our most private issues, we share secrets, we don't judge each other, we know we will face the future together whatever it brings.

ACKNOWLEDGEMENTS

Jeanna: This book would not be complete without one of the kindest, most wonderful women I have known. She was a mom, wife, daughter, and friend. She fought with every tool possible to live. She now resides with our heavenly father, completely healed in Paradise. Her strength and encouragement helped me through some of the darkest days of my life. She blessed my life and the life of anyone who was fortunate enough to know her. Through Jeanna God showed us how true grace, faith, and love should appear. She is missed and loved every day.

Gianetta Reno – You took the chaos I called daily events and notes and turned it into something legible. Your gentle nudging helped me stay focused as we plowed through the many pages of my middle-of-the-night writings. Without you this book might have remained only a dream. Thank you for your dedication, expertise, and consistent belief that this book will help others. I am forever grateful for you.

For the many contributions and resources from:

Memorial Cancer Resource Center

MaryEllen Locher Breast Center

Erlanger Health Systems

Sarah Cannon Cancer Center

Dr. John Gwin

Dr. Brooke Daniel

Marcie Beasley (Nurse Practitioner)

Breast Cancer Support Services of Chattanooga

The Wig Palace

Danna Myatt Photography

Foresight Publishing

"For everyone to whom much is given, from him much will be required."
Luke 12:48 (NKJV)

INTRODUCTION

We all have a story, and there will be a time for all of us when we must choose between ignoring God's voice and desperately begging for His presence. Our story, whatever it may entail, shapes who we are and what we believe. Many would look at my story, what I've gone through over the course of the past few years, and label me as a survivor. Though I do not particularly embrace the term, it pertains for various reasons. But more than anything, I am grateful. Grateful to Jesus for hearing my pleas when I faced the valleys and the shadows; grateful for healing; grateful to be the mother of such a beautiful, loving, strong, and Christ-filled daughter; and grateful to have the opportunity to tell others that regardless of our circumstances He will never leave us.

If you picked up this book, your story might look similar to mine. Maybe you saw on the back of this book that I'm a survivor and you're curious as to how. Or maybe you've been diagnosed yourself and are looking for answers. Well, I don't have all the answers, but I do have experience and resources. Before I was diagnosed with triple negative breast cancer I was like most other moms, very busy. I had worked my way through college and continued my practice beyond graduation. I had earned a Bachelor's in Psychology and a Master's in Clinical Social Work. At the time I was diagnosed, I was teaching adjunct at the university while working on my Doctorate in Education with a concentration in Psychology. I was too busy for needless things such as doctor appointments, as you'll read later when I initially called to cancel the appointment that started this whole journey. Before cancer I was a mother, wife, daughter, business woman, student, teacher, and a mediocre Christian. To this day I am still all of those things, but much stronger in my faith because of the trials and triumphs of cancer.

Unless you have received news such as this, I don't think it's possible to understand how emotionally draining those three words are: "You have cancer." My husband Dan and I had been married nine years and our daughter Alana had just finished second grade. Nothing could have prepared me for that conversation. I ate organic food, worked out on a regular basis, slept in an entirely dark room, and I didn't have any particular habits that would lead to a cancer diagnosis. I had never given much thought to the idea before, and I definitely didn't go through life with the mindset that it would eventually come knocking on my door. When this path opened up in front of me, I couldn't have been more shocked. I can't honestly say I am grateful for the cancer but I am filled with gratitude for the many blessings and positive experiences that came only because of my cancer diagnosis.

I wrote a large portion of this book in the middle of the night, and an even greater portion while going through chemo. As a result, a lot of what I wrote about was fear and worry. I saw the blessings being poured out around me, but my focus was on the diagnosis and the impact it had on our lives. At times I forgot that God is a God of healing regardless of what our well-educated medical community predicts. Thankfully, He isn't limited to healing only certain stages of cancer or any other disease.

When in the midst of suffering our initial response is to question our circumstances. Am I going to die? Why am I going through this? What is happening? How can I have cancer when I feel fine? What did I do to deserve this? It is very difficult to see the larger picture of God's plan when we are trudging through the muck of a life-threatening disease. But James 1:2-4 promises us that the trials and muck we wade through on earth are not for nothing, but for building up our faith. There were many times during my battle with cancer when I couldn't see the whole picture because I was too focused on the chemo treatments and side effects and surgery complications and the all-consuming fear that I would be taken from my daughter. But looking back I can finally see a little clearer that these experiences did produce steadfastness of faith. I am ashamed to say that it took something as drastic as cancer to really force me to depend completely on my Savior. He humbled my spirit. He taught me that my life is to be lived for Him.

It is so easy to look at a story such as mine, with many trials, pain, and uncertainty, and only see the battle. As humans we tend to emphasize the fight more than the victory. But my story isn't just one of struggle, but of hope. There is no story to tell without emphasizing God's role in my emotional and physical recovery. Levi Lusko once said, "Suffering isn't an obstacle, but an opportunity to be used by God," and, therefore, my trial is another person's hope *(Through the Eyes of a Lion, 2015)*.

This book is not only my journey but also what I learned during the past four years. My prayer is that the following words will give hope, encouragement, and help to anyone dealing with any life-altering illness. You'll find everything from questions to ask your medical team to wig care. The resources listed are meant to aid anyone at any stage of treatment. The information within these pages applies to the newly diagnosed, those going through treatment, survivors, and those who love someone with any type of threatening diagnosis. My prayer, in whatever situation you face as you read this book, is that God will use my story to give you hope and encouragement.

- PART I -

Diagnosis

"There is no Goliath ever ahead of you greater than the God who is always in you."
Ann Voskamp

CHAPTER 1

It's Definitely Cancer

Everyone's reaction to a diagnosis is different. A response is neither right nor wrong. The diagnosis and the journey that followed took me from begging God to trusting God. Prior to being diagnosed with breast cancer I was a Christian. My family and I attended church, I taught Sunday School, my daughter and I prayed and read the Bible daily. I believed in God, salvation, and eternity. I had read about faith, thought I completely understood faith, but life had not yet forced me to practice what I studied. Unknowingly, I had not given Jesus full reign in my life. Somewhere in the recesses of thought, I felt I could take care of almost any situation. I was wrong.

Monday, June 11, 2012, began so ordinarily. Alana (my eight-year-old daughter) and I made breakfast as usual then rushed around getting ready for the first day of vacation bible school. After VBS, our friends came over for lunch. As the kids played, I briefly mentioned to my friend that I had a needle biopsy three days earlier. Seeing her concern, I explained I had gone for my routine check-up with my primary care physician the month before and she found a lump in my right breast. She did not believe it was anything of great concern but to be precautionary recommended I see a surgeon for a possible biopsy. I wasn't too concerned since I saw a surgeon annually after learning several years ago I have fibrocystic dense breasts. I told her the surgeon agreed it probably wasn't anything serious but he gave me the option to follow up in a couple of months or have a biopsy to discard all worry. We agreed the biopsy was the best option.

At that time I was working, volunteering at Alana's school, teaching adjunct at the university, and getting my doctorate, all while Alana was in school. Maintaining our family time in the hours after school and before Alana went to bed was priority; sleep was not. I would grade papers and finish up the day's activities long after Alana was asleep. My annual physical was scheduled for May 21, 2012. I called to cancel but the nurse told me it would be a year before I could get another early morning appointment. I kept the appointment. As He has many times in the past, God protected me from my own poor decisions. If I had canceled, the tumor probably would not have been found as early. Later, I would learn how quickly it was growing.

As my friend and I chatted, the phone rang. I fully expected to hear the nurse's voice tell me all was clear. Instead, it was my surgeon. He is a wonderful combination of compassion, knowledge, and skill. I am certain delivering this news was not easy for him. He slowly began to explain something suspicious had shown up on the biopsy report. I asked if it was suspicious or something more. He said, "Well, it's malignant. It's definitely cancer."

As I repeated the news to my friend, the word cancer felt foreign. I felt the tears coming, but knew I could not explain to Alana what I did not understand. I went to my bedroom and stared at my reflection. I thought, "This cannot be happening. I can't have cancer." The woman I saw in the mirror looked healthy.

I shut the door so Alana wouldn't see the breakdown I felt rising. I sat down and sobbed uncontrollably. Images of my daughter flooded my mind. All I could visualize was Alana's beautiful face. Over and over I thought of my precious eight-year-old daughter.

My friend knelt beside me and prayed. She did everything she knew to console me. But the thought that my daughter might grow up without her mommy was unbearable. I thought of my husband and my parents. Negative thoughts and fears consumed me that first hour of the diagnosis.

I wanted desperately to hold Alana but did not want her to see me. I fought back the tears when she came into the room but she knew instantly something was wrong. I told her I wasn't feeling well and that she could go to her swim meet with our friends. She was concerned but content with the answer. She hugged me for a long time before leaving.

After everyone was gone, I sat on the stairs and waited for Dan to get home. I did not want him to hear this news over the phone. As he walked in the door, I collapsed into his arms. Through tears I explained what little I knew. He held me and told me, "Baby, it's going to be okay." In the midst of my despair, his words of reassurance mattered. My parents came over a little later. They certainly did not anticipate the coming news.The look on their faces broke my heart when I explained, "I have cancer." They tried to be strong, to mask their fear. They prayed with me and for me. We tried to talk but eventually sat quietly together waiting for Alana to get home.

Alana and I have always talked openly. I've encouraged her to ask any question or talk about any subject. But this was different. I knew she would be home soon and we had to tell her. I would like to say I used this time to pray for God to give me the words to tell her, but I don't know. My thoughts were a blur of emotions.

When Alana came through the door she instantly knew something was wrong. I held her and explained what little we knew. We held each other as she cried. I tried to assure her I would be okay, that we would all get through this together. Using age appropriate terms, I explained I would need several tests and surgery. I could see the wheels in her eight-year-old mind turning, trying to make sense of her mixed emotions.

This conversation was the first of many. Throughout the surgeries and treatment, Alana would ask questions, give suggestions and participate with my care. We talked about every part of the surgery and chemotherapy. Children know when something is wrong. Most will assume something far worse than reality. Dan and I felt strongly that Alana should be aware of each surgery and what to expect once treatment began.

The days following the diagnosis were emotionally challenging as we dealt with this new reality. I had multiple tests and a core biopsy to determine the type and grade of the tumor. Physically, I felt fine. Emotionally, I struggled with negative thoughts and fears.

Keeping our day-to-day activities as normal as possible was important. Alana continued Taekwondo classes, we cooked, went to swim meets, the grocery store, hiked, went out to dinner, and did all the activities of our normal routine. Alana would ask questions during these days. We talked openly. I tried to answer each question with honesty but without causing fear. The nights were the most difficult. Our evening devotion, prayer, and talks continued, but after Alana would fall asleep I would kneel beside her bed. I begged God to let me live. I begged Him, "Please don't take me from her." I would pray and quietly cry. Some nights I would cry until eventually I was curled on the floor in a fetal position. I wasn't begging for my life because I feared death. The thought of how that might play out had not yet entered my mind. I begged to stay with my daughter.

"So we say with confidence, 'The Lord is my helper; I will not be afraid. What can mere mortals do to me?'"
Hebrews 13:6 (NIV)

"Therefore I tell you, whatever you ask for in prayer, believe that you have received it, and it will be yours."
Mark 11:24 (NIV)

CHAPTER 2

Triple Negative // My Perceived Death Sentence

June 15, 2012, I was meeting with my surgeon to learn the results from the core biopsy and discuss surgery options. Prior to the appointment, the surgery decision was made. I understood we would not know if the cancer was contained until after surgery. I had decided to have a bi-lateral mastectomy. Fortunately, I am blessed with a loving and supportive husband. Dan and I discussed all surgery options prior to the appointment. He said he "wanted me to live and be healthy, that was all that mattered." He and I did as we have for years; we talked in depth but also threw in humor whenever possible. While facing one of the most difficult decisions of my life, I laughed. Dan can make me laugh even in the toughest of times.

My mom, Dan, and a friend, who is an oncology nurse practitioner, waited as my surgeon came into the room. My heart pounded as I waited to hear. He was kind and thorough as he explained the biopsy results. The core biopsy showed the tumor was grade three, invasive, and poorly differentiated. He said it was estimated to be approximately one centimeter but we would not know the stage until after surgery. He went on to explain the cancer had broken through the milk ducts and had grown into the surrounding breast tissue. It was growing quickly and was the highest aggressive grade. Chemotherapy and possibly radiation would follow the surgery. I could feel my body begin to shake but tears did not come.

I learned the three primary hormone receptors for breast cancer are estrogen positive, progesterone positive, and HER2. He said mine was triple negative; it tested negative for all the receptors. In medical terminology "negative" usually refers to something good. I assumed anything with the word negative in it must be good. I had no idea. He said triple negative tends to be more aggressive than the other types of breast cancer. He explained the sentinel node procedure prior to surgery that would tell us if the cancer had spread into the surrounding lymph nodes. Surgery options included lumpectomy, single mastectomy, or a bi-lateral mastectomy. I am sure he explained everything but I had emotionally checked out of the conversation. Normally, I ask questions but not today. We scheduled the surgery for the following week. If possible, I would have had surgery the following day. I wanted this disease out of my body. I knew it was growing, I knew it was aggressive, but I did not know if it was contained to the breast or had spread throughout my body.

Since learning I had breast cancer on Monday, I had hoped and prayed every day that it would be the "mild" type (although I wasn't sure exactly what that meant). I hoped neither chemotherapy nor radiation would be needed, that I could have the surgery, recover, and move on with my life. Everything I learned was opposite to all I had hoped to hear. As we were leaving the office I could feel the anxiety rise. Though it sounds dramatic, I truly feared my heart could stop. We walked back to my surgeon's office. He gave me a prescription to take as needed. It was needed immediately.

As Dan drove me home, I sobbed. I visualized Alana's precious face. How could this happen? Why is this happening? I had waited so long for my baby and now I was going to be taken away from her. I visualized her life, her middle school years, boys, proms, college, marriage, babies, and all the special times a mother wants to share. As these thoughts continued, I looked up and saw the sun was actually shining and cars were all around us, just as any other day. Life around me was continuing as normal but I believed mine was almost over.

I have studied and practiced mental health care but did not fully comprehend a place of complete hopelessness until those moments. I could hear Dan's voice desperately trying to console me. I could feel my mom's hands as she tried to comfort me. I wanted to believe their words but my mind traveled to every dark and irrational place imaginable.

Once home, my mom continued her attempts to console me. She and Dan worked to combat each negative statement. I wanted to believe them but I also understood the possibilities. We are told to "be joyful always; pray continually; give thanks in all circumstances" (I Thessalonians 5:16 NIV). I did none of these.

It never ceases to amaze me how God will use someone else to help us help ourselves. My dad left the room I was in and walked to the kitchen. I'm sure the pain of seeing me so distraught was almost too much for him to bear. A short time later I walked into my kitchen. My dad did not hear me. For a brief moment I saw my dad slumped over, head bent with a look of complete despair. I had never seen him look so discouraged and defeated. I could physically feel his pain. When he realized I was in the room, he quickly sat up appearing strong again. I wrapped my arms around him and, for the first time that day, I spoke positive words. I told him, "Daddy, I will be okay." Though I did not yet believe, those were the words we both needed to hear.

Friday June 15, 2012, was the worst day. I was given what I believed to be a death sentence. Prior to this, I had difficult times but I always knew everything would eventually get better. I no longer had that reassurance. I had never fully relied on Jesus. I knew I could not do this on my own. I had to have Jesus to get my family and me through this journey.

Later that night, after Alana was asleep, Dan and I talked. He held me as I cried and eventually fell asleep. At 2:00 in the morning a friend texted me positive websites she found about triple negative breast cancer (TNBC). She also sent a phone number to a cancer support hotline. I have always encouraged others to reach out for support but I had never followed this advice. At 3:00 AM I called the hotline. The phone call was nothing short of miraculous. Carmen, in California, answered my call. She was a God-given angel to me that night. I told her what little information I knew and, to my surprise, she had been diagnosed with TNBC ten years earlier. We were both astonished. Carmen explained that callers usually have to request for someone who had triple negative (TN) to call them back because it is rarer than the other types. She also said she very seldom answers hotline calls. This was the first time I allowed myself to strongly feel God's presence. He had been with me but I was so preoccupied with begging that I didn't stop to realize He was already there.

During our conversation Carmen described her chemo treatments. She emphasized the importance of rest, exercise, and listening to my body. She wisely suggested I view chemo as an ally. I would later embrace this suggestion and began to change my view of chemo as a toxin to chemo, my collaborator. I saw my first glimmer of hope since the prior day. I could fight cancer alongside the chemo and surgery, something I might not have felt without God using Carmen to help me.

Later that day God again provided hope through two visits with friends. One of my closest friends came with healing cards. Each small card contained a scripture related to healing. She believed strongly that God is still a God of healing and that He wants us to ask and then believe. I would later gain strength knowing her faith in my healing would not waver throughout the long journey ahead. The cards filled with God's words regarding healing and believing would become invaluable to me. Later, another friend came by. He was 32 years old and had gone through multiple rounds of chemotherapy treatment for lung cancer. He was now strong, healthy, and cancer-free. God allowed me to see a living example of healing. These two visits gave me hope that maybe I wasn't going to die. Maybe healing wasn't only in the scriptures; maybe God still healed.

That night I went to a prayer service with my friend who had brought me the healing cards. After the quiet prayer time, one of the ministers asked if they could place oil on my head and pray over me. I am ashamed to admit it, but this was very foreign to me. At first, I was uncomfortable but having a life threatening illness forced me to step out of my area of comfort. If it were not for the diagnosis, I don't know if I would have ever experienced this God-filled moment.

Sunday, June 17, 2012, Dan, Alana, and I went to church. As I walked into our small group class, it was obvious everyone knew. They told me they were all praying for me. I thanked them as God gave me the words to speak. I told them of the week's events, of the uncertainty ahead, the fear, and of my perceived death sentence. God gave me the courage to be transparent when I told them I was, at best, a mediocre Christian. Again, I was ashamed to admit it, but it took a cancer diagnosis for me to completely rely on Jesus. At the end of our time, the class members gathered around me and prayed. Afterward, several people thanked me for being honest and said they too felt mediocre at best. God gave me the courage to speak honestly that Sunday morning. Prior to the cancer diagnosis, I was spiritually quiet. Other than with Alana, I rarely talked in depth about my relationship with God. I had felt that relationship was private, between God and me. I was certainly not comfortable speaking publicly about my struggles, fears, and beliefs. Looking back, I see that Sunday morning as my first opportunity to speak openly about this journey, the necessity of faith, and, most importantly, leaning on Jesus.

"Trust in the Lord with all your heart and lean not on your own understanding; in all your ways submit to him, and he will make your paths straight."
Proverbs 3:5-6 (NIV)

CHAPTER 3

Meet Your Treatment Team

Treatment plans are different just as cancers are different. Yet during a cancer diagnosis you will have what is called a treatment team, a group of doctors, surgeons, and oncology specialists dedicated to your individualized plan. The following are members who could potentially be part of your treatment team depending on your specific needs[1].

NURSE NAVIGATOR:

A diagnosis brings many medical decisions. These decisions will affect your body, your future, your family and friends. Combined with the emotions of learning you have cancer, these important, life-altering decisions are difficult. I encourage anyone going through an illness to work with a nurse navigator. He or she will help you understand your pathology report as you decide your best possible treatment path. You will be faced with a mound of paperwork and test results as information is moved between surgeons, oncologists, and other specialists. Hospitals may refer to this position as a nurse navigator, social worker, case manager, or patient advocate. Working with these professionals can be your personal connection to the many resources within your medical community. A nurse navigator or patient advocate can help you be certain your results are pushed through in a timely manner as you wait for the next step of care.

Your medical team will most likely consist of some or all of the following: your surgeon, oncologist, radiation oncologist, reconstruction specialist, dietitian, and social worker. The care coordinator will act as a liaison between you and each of these professionals, especially in the early days of your diagnosis. In addition to being a liaison among a sea of medical professionals, your nurse navigator can provide emotional support or help alleviate some of your burden by coordinating your treatment while you focus on getting better.

ONCOLOGIST

An oncologist is a doctor who specializes in cancer diagnosis and treatment. He or she will review your pathology report with you and set up your treatment plan. Your oncologist will also perform your follow-up appointments when treatment is complete.

SURGEON

Your surgeon is the doctor who will perform either a lumpectomy or mastectomy to remove the cancer, depending on which surgery you choose.

RECONSTRUCTION SPECIALIST

If you choose to reconstruct your breasts after a mastectomy, you will consult with a reconstruction specialist. This is a surgeon who specializes in rebuilding the breasts after they have been removed.

RADIATION ONCOLOGIST

If part of your treatment plan includes radiation, you will consult with a radiation oncologist. The radiation oncologist is in charge of determining how many rounds of treatment you need and the scheduling of those treatments.

CHEMO NURSE

A chemo nurse will help administer the chemotherapy drugs during each treatment. Depending on your treatment center, you will most likely have a different nurse during each visit.

All of the nurses that administered my treatment were wonderful, knowledgeable, and compassionate. I am forever grateful to all members of my medical team. You continue to provide outstanding care mixed with an unmatched level of compassion.

"Out of suffering have emerged the strongest souls; the most massive characters are seared with scars."
Kahill Gibrar

CHAPTER 4

Questions to Ask Your Treatment Team

This is not a chapter of answers but questions. Immediately after a diagnosis we must schedule an appointment with a surgeon, radiologist, reconstruction specialist, and oncologist. We just learned we have cancer and now we're asked to make decisions quickly that will affect us the rest of our lives. I was given notebooks filled with information but I didn't have the emotional energy to sort through the pages or do the research needed to compile a list of intelligent questions. I wanted a condensed list of the most urgent questions I needed answered during each appointment. The following is that list. These questions are a compilation of the most commonly asked questions from oncologists, surgeons, other medical professionals, my experience, and the American Cancer Society[1 & 2]. If you're recently diagnosed, completed treatment, or in the midst of treatment, these questions will help you understand what to expect immediately and in the future.

It is also very important to remember during your initial visit with each specialist that you will only retain about 10% of the information. Ask a family member or friend to go with you. Take notes to help recall all the details. Once treatment starts, always tell your doctor about any side effects you are experiencing. There are many options to control the side effects of the medications, but your medical team can't help you if they are not aware of your symptoms.

Questions for the doctor before your biopsy
- What type of biopsy will I have?
- How long will the biopsy take?
- Will I be awake or asleep during the biopsy?
- Can I drive home afterward or will I need someone to drive me?
- Where will the scar be? What will it look like?

- How soon will I know the results?
- Do I call you or will you call me with the results?
- Will you or someone else explain the biopsy results to me?

Questions for the oncologist on the initial visit

- What is my diagnosis?
- Will we work to control or cure?
- What are my treatment and/or surgery options?
- What is the expected length of my treatment?
- What is our long-term goal?
- What changes can I make to reduce the risk of recurrence?
- How will treatment reduce the risk of recurrence?

Questions for the oncologist regarding chemo

- Why do I need chemo?
- What is the goal of chemo in my case?
- What drugs will I be taking and why?
- What can I expect if I do not take the treatment?
- How will we know if the chemo is working?
- After chemo, will I be cured or will we work to control the cancer?
- Are there other ways besides chemo to treat my cancer?
- If chemo doesn't work, are there other treatments for me?
- How will the medicine be given (IV, orally, both), how often will I have treatment, and for how long?
- Do I need a chemo port? If so, when?
- Where will I get chemo? Can I visit the chemo room prior to my first treatment?
- Will my hair come out?
- Will I need someone to drive me after a treatment?
- Are there any over-the-counter medications I should avoid?
- Can I take vitamins and supplements? Any I should avoid?
- Can treatment affect my ability to get pregnant? How long after treatment should I wait before trying to become pregnant?
- What are the possible side effects? Should I call you if I have any of these side effects? What if they happen after hours or on the weekend? Is the evening/weekend phone number the same?
- How will we control side effects?
- Do side effects normally progress with each treatment?

- How long will the side effects last?
- What can I do during treatment to help control side effects?
- Will anti-nausea drugs be used? How will these be given?
- Is there anything I should do to get ready for treatment?
- Do I need to see a cardiologist or any other specialist prior to starting treatment?
- Does my insurance pay for chemo? If not, how will I pay?
- What activities (work, exercise, outdoor activities, etc.) can I do during chemo?
- Are there any restrictions on my activities?

Questions for the oncologist after chemotherapy treatment is complete

- When can I go back to doing things I used to do?
- How often will I need to see you?
- Which tests/scans will be done and why?
- Do I need to be on a special diet?
- What should I watch for to know if the cancer comes back?

Questions for the surgeon

- What type of surgery do you suggest and why?
- Will I need more treatment after surgery?
- If I have a mastectomy will I need radiation?
- How long will I be in the hospital?
- Will I have lymph nodes removed? How many?
- What are the chances that I will have arm swelling (lymphedema)?
- What can I do to prevent or reduce the risk of lymphedema?
- What are the symptoms of lymphedema? When should I see a doctor?
- While I'm in the hospital, what should I expect immediately after surgery?
- What will I look like after the lumpectomy or mastectomy? Do you have pictures?
- When I am discharged, who will tell me how to care for my surgical site?
- Will I go home with drains from my surgical site? How many?
- How will my surgical site feel?
- How long will it be before I'm able to start doing my regular work, housework, and leisure activities?
- How long before I can drive?
- What follow-up care will I need?

Questions for the radiologist regarding radiation therapy

- What happens during each visit?
- How many radiation treatments will I need?
- How long will each visit last?
- What are the possible side effects?
- How will we know radiation is working?
- How do I care for my skin during treatment? Are there certain creams or soaps I should use or avoid?
- Should I use deodorant during treatment?
- Will I be able to work during treatment?
- Are there any restrictions on my activities?
- Can I drive after treatment?
- Do I need to avoid sun exposure?
- What type of sunscreen should I use if I'm going to be outside?

Questions to ask the reconstruction specialist regarding breast reconstruction

- What type of surgery do you recommend and why?
- If I choose reconstruction, will that impact my treatment in any way (time, effectiveness, etc.)?
- What are the pros and cons of this surgery?
- May I see photographs of women who have had the same type of reconstruction at several stages (immediately after surgery, after six months, after one year)?
- May I talk with some of your patients about the operation?
- How long will the surgery last?
- How long will I be in the hospital?
- How long is the recovery period after the surgery?
- What will the reconstructed breast look like and feel like (after surgery, after six months, after one year)?
- Will I have any feeling in the reconstructed breast or nipple?
- Do you recommend nipple sparing? Why or why not?
- Is nipple reconstruction done at the same time as the reconstruction?
- What type of implants do you recommend? Why?
- How much will it cost? Is it covered by insurance?

Questions to ask the genetic specialist about genetic testing

If possible, take a list of any type of cancer in your family

- Can I pass a cancer producing gene to my children?
- Are there ways to reduce the risk of passing a gene on to my children?
- Is there a benefit to being tested?
- Which test should I do – BRCA 1, BRCA 2, the BART, any other genetic test?

- PART II -
Surgery

"But He was pierced for our transgressions, He was crushed for our iniquities; the punishment that brought us peace was upon Him, and by His wounds we are healed."
Isaiah 53:5 (NIV)

CHAPTER 5

Mastectomy // My Mantra –
"Thank you, Jesus, for healing!"

I have been asked many times why I chose a bilateral mastectomy rather than a single mastectomy or a lumpectomy. Prior to surgery, we did not know if the cancer was contained but we did know it was aggressive, invasive, and growing rapidly. I want to emphasize there are no right or wrong decisions, only what is best for you. For me, I wanted the disease out of my body as quickly as possible and I knew if I kept any part of either breast the fear of recurrence would be greater. I understood that cancer can return regardless of the surgery choice but, for me, the mastectomy was the best option. I have not regretted that decision.

There are a plethora of surgery options and the decision can be overwhelming. Consider talking with people who have gone through each of the surgery choices. The American Cancer Society offers the Reach To Recovery program, which connects those diagnosed with a survivor. The program will put you in contact with a survivor who has had the surgery or treatment you are considering.

The medical terminology can be confusing when you need to make a life altering decision somewhat quickly. Below is a quick reference to the most commonly performed surgeries following a breast cancer diagnosis[1]:

Breast-conserving surgeries
- **Lumpectomy** – involves removing only the mass and surrounding breast tissue, sometimes also lymph nodes from the underarm
- **Partial Mastectomy** – involves removing the mass and surrounding breast tissue but removes more than a lumpectomy, however less than a full-mastectomy

Mastectomy – involves removing the entire breast
- **Single Mastectomy** – removes only the breast with the mass
- **Bilateral Mastectomy** – removes both breasts

*****

A few days before my surgery, Alana and I talked about the days ahead. She was sad I had to go to the hospital but looking forward to spending a few days with her friends. Knowing she would come to see me every day at the hospital gave her peace. Alana is extremely intelligent and perceptive. She and I talked openly and honestly about the tests, surgeries, and what we could expect while I was recovering. I encouraged Alana to ask questions and always let me know if she didn't understand something and we would talk more about any subject. These conversations were difficult and many times emotional, but I believe knowing where I would be and that she would see me every day helped tremendously as we prepared for my first surgery. She had been flooded with so much information in a short period of time that I had not yet explained exactly what would take place during the surgery. As we were getting ready to go out one morning, she asked, "What is a mastectomy?" I knew I had to explain without terrifying my eight year old daughter. God intervened and gave me the words and humor to lighten the conversation. I explained, in age-appropriate terms, that mommy was going to have both breasts removed. As soon as the words came out I saw the same look of horror come across her face as the day I told her I have cancer. She began to cry but thankfully God gave me humor in that moment to lessen the impact. I said, "It's okay, it just means mommy can go to the pool without a shirt!" She laughed such a God-given laugh at my silly joke. We both laughed. Jesus said there is "a time to weep and a time to laugh" (Ecclesiastes 3:4 NIV). He gave us the gift of laughter we both needed for that difficult conversation.

The internal struggles continued through the days before my surgery but were not as constant. Each day I would read scripture related to healing. I would pray for healing. I gained a little more faith with each passing day. During this time, I was blessed to be surrounded daily by a loving family and wonderful friends. Most would think the night before a major surgery would be filled with last minute preparations; however my house turned into an impromptu party. A few friends stopped by, followed by a few more. Before long my house was filled with laughter, prayer, and praise. Words cannot express the gratitude I have for everyone who rallied around my family and me throughout this week and the many more difficult times ahead.

June 21, 2012 – my surgery day finally arrived. Although it was only ten days from the day I was diagnosed to the day of surgery, it felt much longer. I was ready to have the cancer out of my body. My first memory after surgery is waking in the recovery room desperate to know if the cancer had spread. I asked the nurse repeatedly if she knew the results. She told me she did not. In my drug-induced state of mind, I was convinced she knew but would not tell me. I knew I had to convince her it was okay to tell me. My post-surgery, anesthesia-filled brain thought it was acceptable to pressure this lady into telling me the results. I finally said to her, "I know you know. I can take it. Just please tell me if it spread." Again, she told me she did not know. I have often thought I should go back and apologize to all the recovery nurses.

As I was wheeled from recovery to my room, we passed my surgeon on his way in to see me. I quickly asked him if the cancer was in my lymph nodes, I heard "no," and that's the last I remember. I gave in to the remaining anesthesia and slept. I placed a lot of emphasis on the cancer being or not being in my lymph nodes. I have since met many people who have had positive lymph nodes and are very long-term survivors.

The next day I was sore but walked so much the nurses finally told me I needed to rest. I was relieved the cancer was gone from my body. We learned the tumor was slightly larger than originally thought but considered stage 1. The tumor was no longer growing inside me but my faith in healing was continuing to grow.

The following day, Saturday June 23, began as the previous day. I walked, visited with family and friends, and enjoyed the day. I felt surprisingly well with minimal soreness. That evening when Dan, my IV pole, and I walked to the chapel, I began to feel weak. Before we could return to my room, Dan was holding me up as I struggled to walk. Once back to my room, we assumed I had simply walked too much and was exhausted. He had to work early the next morning so my life-long friend had come into town to stay with me through the night. Dan did not want to leave but I assured him I was just tired.

I grew weaker and the dizziness increased throughout the night. Around 1:00 AM the nurses took a blood sample. My surgeon was not on call that weekend but another filled in his place to eventually order the blood work. The results showed my red blood count was dangerously low. Assuming the numbers could not be correct, the nurse took another sample. The results were the same. They immediately began blood transfusions that continued throughout most of the night. I did not understand the magnitude of what was happening. I was dizzy, sick, and didn't have the energy to ask questions. Thankfully, my friend asked the questions and reassured my fears as the transfusions continued.

When Dan and my parents returned to the hospital, I was feeling better but grew weaker as the day passed. I also realized there was bruising spreading across my chest, back, and arms. I assumed this was normal after a mastectomy. That night the weakness, lightheadedness, and sickness grew worse as my blood count dropped. Again, the nurses took a blood sample and immediately ordered transfusions that continued through most of the night. The following morning, June 25, I felt better. I had definitely had setbacks during the weekend but I was packed and ready to go home. I missed Alana terribly and I wanted to go home and begin recovery. Dan, my mom, my dad, and I were all waiting for the doctor to come in, explain what happened, and dismiss me. Unfortunately, this was not what happened. When my surgeon came, he knew immediately something was wrong. He explained the severe bruising was caused by hematomas. The blood was building up in the tissue causing my red count to drop and the discoloration to continue. The incisions would need to be reopened to remove the hematomas. He asked how long had it been since I last ate. I remember looking at my dad, mom, and Dan as I struggled to fully understand. I could see the look of fear and shock on their faces as they too worked to comprehend. Two days later I went home. My expected short stay was now a week.

I truly believe Jesus healed me during the surgery. But there were still many moments following the surgeries that I felt afraid or worried the cancer was still looming within. To combat those fears I spoke to my Healer. I have prayed silently for years but for the first time in my Christian life I spoke out loud to God. Years of studying mental health left me reserved to speak out loud when alone but since the diagnosis that reservation was gone. When struggling with fear I would say, "Thank you, Jesus, for my healing." I spoke these words even when I doubted their truth. I learned just saying them gave me the reassurance I needed to get through the moment. If you are struggling with doubt and fear find your mantra of hope then continue to speak the words even if you doubt their truth. Saying words out loud gives them a power they may never have if they remain only in our thoughts. I continue to declare this mantra each time I feel fear or doubts begin to creep in.

"You gain strength, courage, and confidence by every experience in which you really stop to look fear in the face. You must do the thing which you think you cannot do."
Eleanor Roosevelt

CHAPTER 6

What to Expect After Surgery //
The Human Octopus Phase

From lumpectomy to bilateral mastectomy breast cancer surgery is a vital part of the treatment plan. It is a major surgery, and as any major surgery, you will need adequate recovery time. Below are a few things to look out for and expect as you return home from surgery[3 & 4].

Prepare for Recovery – If possible, try to arrange ahead of time tasks that will need to get done while you are recovering from surgery. Ask a spouse, family member, or friend to help with meals, arrange for school drop off and pick up if you have children, and schedule all of your appointments far enough out that you won't be pressured to do too much too fast.

Drains – After a mastectomy one of the biggest surprises coming home from surgery can be dealing with the drainage tubes that are now dangling from your chest. The tubes have bulbs on the end to collect any fluid from the surgical site and keep it from gathering in the wound, which could create an infection. These long tubes and bulbs can almost make you feel like a human octopus with tentacles hanging out from under your clothes. To hide the drains when you go out, you can pin them to the inside of your shirt or to the camisole you will most likely need to wear. Your doctor will instruct you how to empty your drainage bulbs and measure the fluids. You will do this a few times a day (as your doctor instructs) and take note of the amount and appearance of the fluid. Drains are typically removed around two weeks after surgery.

Phantom Pain – During recovery you may experience tingles or sensations in your chest known as "phantom pain." When you have surgery to remove breast cancer, your brain continues to send signals throughout your body, only the signals that once were received by the breast tissue are no longer picked up because they're reconnecting. As a result you might feel something like an itch, pressure, or simply a weird sensation. These feelings will go away as your chest begins to heal.

Limited Movement – Because you have just had major surgery on a part of your body that contains muscles used for most upper-body movement, you will have limited range of motion during recovery. You will regain most of this over time, but during this period your strength and range can be compromised as the components inside your chest begin reconnecting and healing.

Arm Exercises – After surgery your doctor might give you a list of recommended arm exercises to practice daily, especially if you also had lymph nodes removed. These exercises are to help prevent lymphedema from forming in the arm on the side of the surgery, whether it's a lumpectomy on one side or a bi-lateral mastectomy. Lymphedema is when tissues in your body, such as in your arm, swell due to lymph fluid buildup. Though you will have a limited range of motion, try to do these exercises as often as directed by your physician to keep the lymph in your arm from building up and swelling.

REST – You just went through a major surgery, your body needs to regain strength. Ease back into your activities, being mindful of the surgical site as it continues to slowly heal. Remember you will return to cooking, cleaning, laundry, and all those fun activities soon enough.

I emphasize this last point because I did not follow this instruction often enough. I tried with all my strength to continue life as normal. I wanted my "before cancer" daily life back so badly that I did everything possible to maintain that previous lifestyle. That was a mistake. In hindsight, I should have rested more often. Remember, this time is truly a balancing act; be as active as your body will allow but know you will also need extra rest during this recovery phase.

"What lies behind us and what lies before us are tiny matters compared to what lies within us."
Ralph Waldo Emerson

CHAPTER 7

Understanding Your Pathology Report

The pathologist analyzes your biopsy samples and details everything observed under the microscope. Because these reports are written by medical professionals for medical professionals, you may not understand all of what is listed or how it is relevant to you. Understanding your pathology report is important not only for your own knowledge but it is also vital in making key treatment decisions.

Below is a breakdown of the terminology you might see on your pathology report, followed by the definition of each term [5 & 6].

Diagnosis/Final Diagnosis – This is the pathologist's conclusion of your diagnosis and the type of cancer.

Tumor Size – Tumor size is measured in centimeters. The pathologist can estimate the size based on the biopsy sample, but the true size cannot be determined until surgery. Size is one factor in determining the stage of cancer and necessary treatment, but it does not tell the whole story as differentiation (i.e. growth speed) is another important factor.

Non-Invasive vs. Invasive – Like tumor size, whether the tumor is non-invasive or invasive cannot be definitively determined until surgery. When a tumor is *non-invasive* it is "in situ," which means it has not spread outside the milk ducts/lobules where it started. If a tumor is *invasive* it has spread from the original site to surrounding breast tissue and potentially lymph nodes and other parts of the body.

Tumor Grade – Tumor grade is the shape of the cancer cells (i.e. the abnormal cells) in comparison to normal breast tissue cells. The more familiar cancer cells look to normal cells, the lower the grade and vice versa. There are three grades:

- **Grade 1** – well-differentiated (growing slowly), looks most similar to normal cells
- **Grade 2** – moderately-differentiated, between very normal and abnormal
- **Grade 3** – poorly-differentiated (growing quickly), cells are extremely abnormal to normal cells

Hormone Receptor Status – This refers to the proteins found on the outside of the cancer cells that attract certain hormones to help the cancer cells grow. There are two protein receptor types: **estrogen** and **progesterone**. If one of these is present, the cancer is labeled positive for that hormone. For example, Estrogen Positive Breast Cancer (ER positive).

HER2 Status – Human epidermal growth factor receptor 2 (aren't you glad it's just called HER2?!) is a protein that appears on the surface of breast cells and controls their growth and division. But in 25% of cancer cases, these cells grow and divide uncontrollably fast, resulting in breast cancer. If a breast cancer has amplified HER2 genes it is said to be HER2-positive. There are targeted treatments for HER2-positive breast cancer.

Triple Negative – If a tumor is negative for estrogen receptors, progesterone receptors, and HER2, it is deemed triple negative.

Cancer Stage – Cancer stage is based on the varying features of the cancer and helps organize them into categories to best understand a patient's prognosis, determine the best treatment plan, and describe the cancer in a way that can be understood and compared. This a condensed listing of each stage:

- **STAGE 0** – non-invasive breast cancer

- **STAGE 1A**
    - the tumor is up to 2 centimeters *AND*
    - there is no evidence of abnormal cells in the lymph nodes

- **STAGE 1B**
    - there are small groups of cancer cells in the lymph nodes between 0.2 and 2 millimeters (no tumor in the breast) *OR*
    - there is a tumor in the breast no bigger than 2 centimeters and small groups of cancer cells in the lymph nodes between 0.2 and 2 millimeters

- **STAGE 2A**
    - there is cancer larger than 2 millimeters in 1-3 underarm lymph nodes or in lymph nodes near the breastbone (no tumor in the breast) *OR*
    - the tumor is 2 centimeters or smaller and has spread to underarm lymph nodes *OR*
    - the tumor is between 2 and 5 centimeters and is not present in the underarm lymph nodes

- **STAGE 2B**
  - the tumor is between 2 and 5 centimeters and small groups of cancer cells between 0.2 and 2 millimeters are present in the lymph nodes *OR*
  - the tumor is between 2 and 5 centimeters and the cancer has spread to 1-3 underarm lymph nodes or lymph nodes near the breastbone *OR*
  - the tumor is larger than 5 centimeters but is not present in the underarm nodes

- **STAGE 3A**
  - there is either no tumor or a tumor of any size in the breast, and cancer is in 4-9 underarm lymph nodes or lymph nodes near the breastbone *OR*
  - the tumor is larger than 5 centimeters and small groups of breast cancer cells between 0.2 and 2 millimeters are in the lymph nodes *OR*
  - the tumor is larger than 5 centimeters and cancer has spread to 1-3 underarm lymph nodes or lymph nodes near the breastbone

- **STAGE 3B**
  - *inflammatory* breast cancer includes certain physical features found in Stage 3B such as the breast appearing swollen, feeling warm, and the skin reddened.
  - there is a tumor of any size present and cancer has spread to the chest wall and/or skin of breast causing swelling/ulcer *AND*
  - cancer may have spread to up to 9 underarm lymph nodes *OR*
  - cancer may have spread to lymph nodes near breastbone

- **STAGE 3C**
  - the cancer has spread to 10 or more underarm lymph nodes *OR*
  - the cancer has spread to lymph nodes above or below the collarbone *OR*
  - the cancer has spread to underarm lymph nodes or lymph nodes near the breastbone

- **STAGE 4**
  Also known as *advanced* or *metastatic* breast cancer
  - the cancer has spread outside the breast to other organs

Tumor Margins – The rim of the breast tissue surrounding the tumor is known as the tumor margin. These margins are used to determine if all the cancer is removed during surgery. There are three margin descriptions:

- *Negative (Clear) Margins* – margins do not contain cancer cells
- *Positive (Involved) Margins* – margins contain cancer cells, more treatment is necessary
- *Close Margins* – cancer cells approach, but do not touch, the edge of the tissue, more treatment might be necessary

Lymph Node Status – To determine how many lymph nodes are removed, doctors will use a *Sentinel Node Dye* test. The dye injected into lymph nodes will highlight the leading node, called the sentinel node. Doctors will then remove that node and surrounding nodes (the number of nodes removed will vary).

*****

This chapter was added after researching the medical terminology most often used during a breast cancer diagnosis. My hope is that this reference gives a quick understanding of terms that don't always make sense when we're attempting to understand what is happening within our bodies. It's also important to keep a copy of your original pathology report. This will come in handy if you decide to get a second opinion or want to review your results years after your diagnosis. You can read more about second opinions in chapter 12.

"Anxiety in a man's heart weighs it down, but an encouraging word makes it glad."
Proverbs 12:25

CHAPTER 8

Weeks Leading up to Chemo Treatment // The Road to Chemo

Once home from the hospital, my mom or I would drain and measure the amount of blood and fluid draining into the tubes at each incision site. The amount drained determined when the tubes could be removed. Shortly after surgery, I also developed an infection and a fluid pocket at one of the drain sites. My surgeon drained the fluid pocket and treated the infection before chemo began. The drainage tubes were cumbersome but I would pin them under my shirt and hope they didn't slip out. During one of my first adventures out after surgery, I noticed someone trying to discreetly look down toward my waist as we talked. I quickly realized one of the fluid tubes had slipped and was dangling outside my shirt. I could only imagine what they were thinking so I laughed and explained that was a "left over" souvenir from my recent surgery.

The days following surgery were filled with family and friends. Dan, my parents, and my aunt rarely left my side. I was amazed at the generosity and love we received from everyone. My sister and niece cleaned my house. My niece and her husband bought my one and only "Sharon pizza." We spent countless hours together. We ate together, watched movies together, and truly enjoyed spending time with each other. I'll never know what other plans they gave up or changed during this time but all that seemed to matter was being together as a family. I am forever grateful for this time.

I am so blessed to have not just one but two wonderful families. Dan's family is my family. Most refer to their spouse's family as their "in-laws." For us, this does not apply. They came to see us almost daily bringing food and anything we could possibly need or want. We ate, laughed, prayed, and enjoyed every minute of our time together. I've often thought James (5:16) must have known my mother-in-law when he wrote "the prayer of the righteous is powerful and effective." She is truly one of the most righteous, Christ-filled women I have known.

After surgery it would be about a month before I started chemo. I wished many times that surgery was the last of this process. However, I continued to feel strongly that God wanted me to walk this path for a reason. I began writing shortly after I was diagnosed. I wrote of the fear, the physical and emotional pain, the frustration, and the joy (yes, joy) that comes from this diagnosis. Each peak and valley on this roller coaster of emotions was more intense than I knew possible.

During these weeks after surgery and before treatment began, we did all our usual routine of activities. My range of motion was limited and the soreness continued but I was recovering more each day. I had to work daily, sometimes hourly, to control my thoughts. When I gave the fear to Jesus I felt peace. When I allowed fear to control, all peace was gone. Emotions could jump from joy and peace to fear and anxiety with one runaway thought. These thoughts can come when you least expect them, as they did while Alana and I were at a bridal shower. We were enjoying the party and everything was fine but as we watched the bride-to-be open her gifts, the thoughts came quickly and unexpectedly: "Would I be here for Alana's bridal shower?" "Would I be here for her wedding?" "Would I even be here for her 9th birthday?" To everyone around me I appeared normal but internally I was filled with anxiety. I went to the bathroom and prayed. I apologized for my lack of faith and, again, thanked Jesus for my healing. I felt as the father did in Mark 9:24: "Lord I believe; please help my disbelief."

July 19, 2012, Dan and I had our first meeting with my oncologist. Prior to the meeting, we had lunch and walked through a few of my favorite shops. The thought ran through my mind again how "normal" we must appear, but life was not normal, at least not the normal I once knew. I had my list of questions and was ready to face this next phase of my journey. Once we arrived at the oncology office, we sat quietly as we waited to meet this important member of my treatment team. Neither one of us knew what to expect, but she immediately made us feel comfortable. She explained the goal with any cancer diagnosis is to cure or control. She said surgery removed the tumor but, because the cancer was aggressive and growing rapidly, a cancerous cell or cells could have escaped. She said because the cancer was aggressive, treatment would need to be aggressive. I would need four treatments of Adriamycin and Cytoxan, also known as the Red Devil (I would later understand why), followed by twelve treatments of Paclitaxel. My oncologist went

July 21, 2012 It's only 11:00 a.m and already a great day! Alana's friends are here and we've laughed, played games and danced. my life is so great! I love my life! please God let me live!

over possible side effects and medications to counter side effects. She explained my pathology report, and went on to tell me without chemo I had approximately 30% chance of recurrence but with chemo I could reduce that chance to 15%. My first treatment was scheduled for the following week.

Two days before chemotherapy began I had a chemo port surgically inserted into the left side of my chest. The port was a small plastic disc that connected to a large vein. The chemotherapy drugs would be given through a small needle that fit into the top of the device. During and after treatment they would access the port to draw blood and administer fluids. While this was a physical symbol that reminded me of my cancer journey, I did manage to find a little humor as time went on (it's all in how you look at it). When my top would slightly move, exposing the odd round object protruding from my chest, I would see some of the most humorous facial expressions. I can only imagine what people thought as they glimpsed the weird looking device bulging from my chest. Sometimes I explained, other times I left it to the imagination.

After the procedure, the nurse took us to the chemo infusion room (I recommend visiting your treatment room before starting chemo). As I surveyed the room, I again was consumed with the reality that this was really happening. I thought, "I had cancer, there are tubes sticking out of my body, and now I'm facing the very real possibility of being very sick." After a cancer diagnosis, life changes quickly and emotions can struggle to keep up with the rapid changes. It had been over a month since my diagnosis but, at times, the entire experience still felt as though I might wake from a bad dream.

To combat the cancer haze, it's a good idea to have questions prepared when meeting with your oncologist and treatment team members. Having your questions ready ahead of time will give you a guide, almost like a script, for those moments when you're face-to-face with the medical world and slip into surreal mode. Chapter 4 lists those important questions to discuss with your oncologist, surgeon, and the rest of your treatment team.

The next day, my parents and I went over all the information from the oncologist. I spoke evenly, only stumbling as I spoke of the chance of recurrence. I have often thought how terrible all this must be for them. As a mom, I cannot imagine how terrified I would be in their place. I knew they were scared, but they always appeared strong for me. Their support and encouragement never wavered. I am blessed beyond words to have such amazing parents.

- PART III -
Treatment

*"Anxiety weighs down the heart, but
a kind word cheers it up."*
Proverbs 12:25 (NIV)

CHAPTER 9

Encouragement for the Chemo Bound

For many years I have believed in the importance of both traditional and holistic approaches to health, prevention, medication, and treatment. Prior to this diagnosis, if someone had asked if I would take chemotherapy or choose a more natural path, I am uncertain what that answer would have been.I've heard people say, "If I am ever diagnosed with cancer, there is no way I will do chemo." I now know this is not a decision you can possibly make until faced with the multitude of decisions, information, research, advice (wanted and unwanted), and the fear that accompanies a traumatic diagnosis.

During treatment I read an article from a physician that practiced only natural forms of medicine. Though I stopped reading the article because I felt it could cause me to second guess my decision to take chemo, I read enough to know the article focused only on negative side effects of traditional treatment. The article spoke of the risks of treatment, emphasizing the risks as not worth the reduction in the statistical probability of recurrence. Contrary to this, I believe it is an individual decision that must be made after much prayer, research, and conversation. When I was forced to make this decision I chose, without hesitation, to pursue the traditional route of treatment.

Most of us facing chemo are hesitant because of the onslaught of negative information. Chemo drugs do kill cancer cells, but they can also kill healthy cells too. These healthy cells are usually the ones that reproduce quickly, like hair cells and the cells in your mouth, which can lead to hair loss and possibly mouth sores[2]. Both are nasty side effects that I experienced first-hand.

I began chemo with a combination of drugs known as the Red Devil. During those four rounds of Adriamycin and Cytoxan (A/C) I suffered, but there were also stretches of time that were free of side effects. After completing the A/C treatment, I began twelve rounds of another chemo known as Paclitaxel. Thankfully, the side effects were minimal with this drug compared to the A/C.

Chemo serves many purposes in the fight against cancer. Different chemotherapy drugs can be combined to more effectively kill cancer cells and may even be combined with other treatments like radiation. Typically chemo is given through a port in the chest, but there are also other methods of administering the drugs. The most common uses of chemo include[2]:

- To keep the cancer from spreading
- To make the cancer grow slower
- To kill cancer cells that may have spread to other parts of the body
- To make side effects from cancer better
- To cure cancer

In the words of J.R.R. Tolkien, "Faithless is he that says farewell when the road darkens" (*Fellowship of the Ring*, 1954). Don't turn away because the chemo road looks grim and dark. There is light on the other end. It takes strength and courage to get there, but continually ask for both from our Heavenly Father. Remember we are not alone in the fight. While chemo gives you a chance to fight off the enemy cells, the Lord takes up arms as well: "The Lord will fight for you; you need only be still" (Exodus 14:14 NIV). God doesn't stand idle while we suffer; He is active in the fight. We must continually trust in His power and His faithfulness. Cancer and the treatment that follows is a journey and it is a struggle. But you will never be alone. Have faith the Lord will be your light and protector as you walk through the path of chemotherapy.

"Attitude is a little thing that makes a big difference."
Winston Churchill

CHAPTER 10

Chemotherapy Basics

CHEMOTHERAPY MUST HAVE'S

Below is a list of items that will be helpful during chemo treatments.

- Sweater or jacket—it is always cold in the chemo room
- Blanket—some people take a blanket but I used the blankets provided
- Comfortable clothing—but keep in mind the nurses need to easily access your port (I forgot and wore a turtleneck sweater to my first treatment)
- Book, tablet, phone, magazines, laptop, journal, or other items to pass the time
- Knitting, sewing, other craft projects (I never did any of these but I admire those who can)
- Headphones—if you want quiet time use them even if you're not listening to anything
- Water or other drinks, lunch or snacks (my mom packed our lunch for each treatment)
- Lip balm and hand cream
- Gum, hard candy, mints—especially if you "taste" the medication as it goes through your port

TAKING CARE OF YOURSELF DURING CHEMO[2]

- Hydrate, hydrate, hydrate! Having fluids in your system helps reduce aches, nausea, and simply makes everything in your body work better. Most chemo rooms are closed on the weekends so if I was aching or nauseous I would get my fluids "topped off" on Friday.
- Rest up. Chemo can take a toll on your body, be sure to give yourself plenty of time to relax during treatment (sometimes easier said than done, especially when you have young children).

- Eat healthy foods as much as possible. Nutrition during treatment is vital to keep your body fueled well. See chapter 15 for more information on nutrition during and after treatment.
- Stay active as much as possible. Exercise helps reduce stress, fatigue, and appetite changes caused by the treatment. Be sure to check with your doctor on what activities are approved.
- Ask your doctor about alcohol during treatment. Some alcohol can interfere with certain chemo drugs, so check with your doctor before that big party.
- Tell your doctor all the vitamins and supplements you take. Some vitamins and supplements can counteract certain chemo drugs. For example, I was told Vitamin C supplements could reduce the effectiveness of treatment.
- Keep your mind focused on the treatment goal. Positive thinking positively impacts behavior and health (see chapter 20 for more information on mind-body connection).

Roxanne Brown wrote an excellent resource book for those facing chemo titled *Chemo: Secrets to Thriving*. My first thought when I read the title was, "I'm barely surviving much less thriving." Don't let the title mislead you, the book provides many resources and tips for those beginning or in treatment[7].

- See your gynecologist for your annual exam—this would be a good time to discuss fertility and future pregnancy questions with your doctor if this applies to you
- Purchase at least one wig or find a boutique with donated wigs (see chapter 13 for more hair info)
- Have your teeth cleaned
- Stop anti-oxidant supplements
- Have your skin checked for suspicious moles (the freckle's ugly cousin)
- Talk with your doctor if you're struggling with anxiety or sleeplessness
- Remind any medical personnel before treatment, blood draws, or blood pressure checks if you've had lymph nodes removed

Above all, talk with your doctor about taking care of these items before you begin chemo and always tell him/her before beginning or stopping any medications or supplements.

"Pain insists upon being attended to. God whispers to us in our pleasures, speaks in our consciences, but shouts in our pains. It is His megaphone to rouse a deaf world."
C.S. Lewis, The Problem of Pain

CHAPTER 11

First Chemo Treatment //
Dancing with the Red Devil

As I describe my experience with chemotherapy, I want to emphasize that my experiences will not necessarily be yours. I took sixteen chemotherapy treatments—four rounds of Adriamycin and Cytoxan (A/C) and twelve rounds of Paclitaxel. The following are my experiences but are certainly not indicative of all who take chemotherapy.

July 25, 2012, Dan was beside me as the nurse hooked the IV to the port in my chest. She asked if I wanted the area numbed before she started the chemo. This was all such a bizarre feeling. As the drugs entered my body, the nurse knelt beside me and explained what would most likely happen over the next couple of weeks. A few tears fell as she reminded me I only had about two more weeks before my hair started to come out. I dreaded losing my hair and all the sickness that might come, but I knew this path was necessary.

Treatment went through most of the day. I wrote notes for this book as I sat quietly in my "chemo chair." Thankfully I did not have a reaction to either chemo drug. After treatment, I felt surprisingly good and even stopped for dinner on the way home. I thought I would make it through the evening unscathed, but then the sickness came. The nausea was so severe I could not get relief. I threw up multiple times throughout the night. I learned a very valuable lesson: if you are taking drugs that have a high probability of making you sick, you should not eat salmon. Let's just say that was not a good experience.

The sudden reaction I had to the chemo was not the norm. Though the A/C treatment is known to be extremely difficult, most people do not experience a reaction that soon. I do not want the description of my side effects to be considered typical. Reactions to chemo treatments vary depending on the type of drug and the patient's body. I get nauseated easily. I was nauseated during my pregnancy, I get nauseated on car trips, I can get nauseous turning my head too quickly (okay, that could be a slight exaggeration). But, as you will see in the chapters to come, I experienced intense side effects. I hope these experiences show that extreme circumstances can (eventually) produce perseverance and hope. "We also rejoice in our suffering, because we know that suffering produces perseverance; perseverance, character, and character, hope" (Romans 5:3-4 NIV). I wish I could write I rejoiced in the suffering but I did not. I had a few pity parties, but each time I would (eventually) pray and ask for the strength to continue.

The following day my mom came as she would throughout the most difficult days. That first week brought pain in places I didn't know could hurt. It hurt to open and close my eyes. My hair hurt. My entire body ached. I stayed in bed most of the first day. The second day I was slightly better and was able to muster enough strength to take a shower. My friend took Alana and me to the oncology center for more IV anti-nausea medicine and fluids. The meds helped a little but the sickness was still overwhelming. I took the pain pills to help with the body aches but the pain came in full force the third day. I stayed in bed most of the day. I was nauseated, constipated and could not eat or sleep. Every part of my body hurt. I truly thought I would possibly be sick a couple of days and then bounce back. I had not expected the pain and nausea to be so severe. "When will this get better?" "Will I ever feel normal again?" I had been in bed all morning, most of the time crying. I wasn't sure if my expectations had been too high or if I was just one of the unlucky ones who couldn't find relief.

The next day (day four) every inch of my body hurt and the nausea wasn't getting better. I wanted desperately to have my previous life back and spend the day with Alana. I knew this would not be possible but, thankfully, my friends made sure Alana's day went on as normal as possible. Our neighbor picked her up to go to the pool and, as they drove past our house, I watched as she stared intently out the window. I cried wondering what she was thinking. Is she more worried than I realize? Is she more scared than I know? Is she relying on God? Am I relying on God? I felt physically and emotionally miserable as I returned to bed.

Later that night as Alana and I talked and prayed, I again asked God to give me the strength to get through the coming months. I didn't know what the weeks and months ahead would bring, but falling asleep with her sweet little hand in mine gave me the comfort and peace I needed in that moment.

The next day I felt slightly better, at least well enough to move from the bed to the sofa. As always, if we look for them, there will be many bright moments even in the weakest times. Alana was spending the night at a friend's house, Dan was at work, and my mom came to keep me company. I was beginning to feel closer to normal than I had in days. Nothing extraordinary happened. Mom and I sat quietly and watched a movie. I couldn't remember the last time we watched a movie together, we were usually running errands or on the go. I learned to treasure the most ordinary of events.

The sixth day after treatment the nausea wasn't as severe and the pain had lessoned. My mother-in-law, sister-in-law, and niece brought Alana, mom, and I lunch. As we sat around the table I thought of the tremendous influence and help each of these women had been since the diagnosis. They would do anything for us and never stopped praying. I am thankful to have a community of strong Christian women surrounding Alana and me. After any type of life-altering illness these uneventful, quiet moments become some of the most cherished memories. I never appreciated "normal" so much until I lost it.

*****

Be aware of what you read. I certainly don't always practice this sound advice, but I highly recommend weeding through the negative information readily available online. If possible, have a friend or family member pre-read information, especially during the initial stages of a diagnosis. I avoided my computer, using it only to grade papers and submit grades. I was fearful of what I might read. There were times when I felt I could be one negative statistic away from a complete breakdown. The second week after my first treatment I encountered what I had tried to avoid— frightening statistics about triple negative breast cancer (TNBC). These numbers are not difficult to find. I stumbled onto the statistics as I was reading an article regarding a treatment being used for TNBC. Skimming the article, I was intrigued by the information until the dreaded fact appeared. I read it before I realized. I had avoided this type of information for the past month and there it was, glaring off the page. I waited for the fear but it didn't come. I cannot say I wasn't impacted by the statistic, but I was not overwhelmed. I felt surprisingly calm. The peace that swept over me was without a doubt the presence of God. As I read the article, God wrapped His arms around me and soothed my fears. He intervened and I was actually excited to have the opportunity to see how He would use my journey to help others (and me) understand His love and His powerful gift of healing. God placed confidence in my heart that night that those numbers did not pertain to me. Regardless of the information, I was not a statistic.

We are not a number. We are individuals. That statistical probability does not take into consideration faith, lifestyle, outlook, or attitude. A statistic is a generalization and many times if you go back to the original source you'll find that some statistics aren't as credible as others. When I was diagnosed with TNBC, some of the literature talked of the "rare and extremely aggressive" nature of triple negative. The information gave the disease power, even nicknaming it "the killer of young women" and "beastly." Most adjectives used were fear-inducing descriptions. While we cannot blind ourselves to the reality that bad things happen in the fight against cancer, we can't put our necks on the chopping block solely because of numbers. Instead of focusing on the negatives of my diagnosis, I concentrated on the research showing how well triple negative responds to chemo.

*****

After recovering from the first week of treatment, I felt good. I was back to all normal daily activities. Two weeks following the first treatment I went to my oncologist's office for my weekly blood count. I felt tired but good. Mom, Alana, and I had plans for the day but were forced to cancel after being told my white cell count was extremely low and I had a fever of 100.4. The nurse said I would have to be admitted to the hospital if my temperature reached 100.5. I was astonished that I could feel so good and still be sick. We returned home after picking up my prescriptions. Throughout the evening I checked my temperature, each time worried that the mere tenth of a degree would appear and I would have to go to the hospital. At 8:30 PM the thermometer read 101.6. My aunt and I started packing my bag to go to the hospital. As we were leaving, the doctor called to tell me he could prescribe a strong antibiotic that could potentially keep me from being hospitalized. I told him I would try anything. Thankfully, the antibiotic and Tylenol reduced the fever and I was able to stay home.

During this time I noticed my throat was sore but nothing severe. In hindsight my temperature was probably rising as an indicator of the throat abscesses that were starting to form. At the time I had no idea I was about to endure the worst pain since my diagnosis. Over the next two days, the pain worsened. I went to the chemo lab but both the doctor and nurses were uncertain what was causing the pain. They said to continue the antibiotic and the prescribed "miracle mouthwash" but the pain was becoming unbearable. My throat felt like an open blister; the pain intensified each time I swallowed. By the second night the pain was so severe it had spread into my right ear.

Dan begged me to go to the ER. I was crying and suffering so much he didn't know what to do. He felt so helpless he sat beside me and cried. I called my oncologist's office and they recommended I go to the emergency room. I prayed for any relief.

Once in the hospital, I was given enough medication that I could eventually rest. But as soon as the IV pain medication was stopped and I was released, the pain returned. I don't always take prescription pain meds as often as directed but this time I took them every few hours as the doctor had prescribed. The pain continued over the next couple days but the medication kept it somewhat manageable

August 7, fourteen days after my first treatment and while still managing the throat pain, Alana and I were going to school to register for third grade. While getting ready to leave that morning, I brushed through my hair and quickly realized I was holding a large handful of hair. I sat in the bathroom and cried. I didn't want Alana to know yet so I quietly called Dan. He assured me it was no big deal to be bald. I told him that was easy for him to say, he had been bald for ten years. Thankfully, my husband was not threatened by the fact that we would soon have matching heads. The nurses had told me what to expect, I had read about hair loss, I knew this would happen but I was sad. Somewhere deep inside I think we all hope to be that one in a million who doesn't lose their hair. I was not.

Prior to starting chemo, Alana and I talked about my hair coming out. We laughed at the thought of both her parents being bald. I was determined to make this a fun memory. I did not want Alana to be sad but rather enjoy this opportunity to be an eight-year-old hairdresser! We decided she would cut and style my hair any way she wanted and then shave my head.

August 2012 It's 2:15 a.m. my throat feels like a giant open blister. It brings tears to my eyes just to swallow. The pain is horrible! When I swallow the pain is so bad it's going into my right ear. I miss Alana. I want her home and I want us to do all the things we did before cancer. I want the pain to go away.

August 12 was a beautiful, clear day. We set up a salon on our deck, complete with spray bottles, spray conditioner, combs, and salon scissors to make it official. I put on a vampire cape I had used for Halloween to serve as my salon cape and sat in the chair ready for my new look. She would cut my hair any way she wanted. We laughed, talked, and took funny pictures as she created my new look. There were no tears, only laughter. Our back deck is private, so we were able to keep this moment just between the two of us. Alana shaving my head gave us an opportunity to take a bad situation and turn it into a fun day, a memory Alana and I will always cherish. After all, it's not every day that a child gets to cut their mom's hair!

I highly recommend including your children in this phase of treatment. Kids will have a blast doing whatever they want with your hair. How many times do they have an opportunity to cut and style your hair in any crazy way they desire? Probably not many, so take advantage of this time together. Yes, it was difficult to accept I was losing all my hair but it was much more important to make this a good memory for Alana. You can read more hair tips and information in chapter 13.

The following day I arrived at the oncologist office for my second treatment with my (borrowed) wig and freshly shaved head. The throat pain continued but, most of the time, was manageable with medication. When my oncologist came in the room I knew immediately something was wrong. My blood count was low and the infection in my throat was severe. She said treatment would have to be postponed and she sent me immediately to an Ear Nose and Throat specialist. Because the recommended physician was out for the day, the office sent me to another doctor in the group. I do not often make negative remarks about providers, but this was an exception. Once in the chair, he put four shots directly into one of the abscessed ulcers in my throat and then proceeded to lance (AKA cut) a hole into the abscess …without medication or anesthesia! The pain was unbearable. I pushed his hand out of my mouth and told him to stop. No one should go through that procedure without sedation.

He told me I would need a CT scan if the abscesses didn't improve to rule out the possibility of this being a new cancer. I knew, even with my tendency to worry, this was not a new cancer. The pain had come quickly and fiercely after a chemo treatment. It was a rare side effect. My mom and I left the office stunned by the comments but thankful it was over.

The pain continued to lessen over the next few days. The chemo-induced tonsillar ulcers may have grown because I didn't have the Neulasta injection after my first treatment. Neulasta is a drug oncologists typically give within 24 hours of an A/C chemo treatment. Since I was young and otherwise healthy, we decided to try the first treatment without the drug. I took the injection following the next three A/C treatments.

I often look back on my experiences and remember questioning why I had to go through some of the side effects of this disease and its treatment. I was unable to see the purpose behind the suffering when in the midst, but now I can clearly see how God was aligning His plans during this time. He was building an opportunity to encourage others while also changing my mindset. I learned delaying a treatment or having the strength of the drugs reduced is somewhat common. After the infection, the chemo was reduced to 80% of the original strength. If my throat abscesses hadn't been so severe, I probably would have argued to continue the chemo full force. Though my experience was difficult, God's purposes and comforts were ever present throughout: *"Praise be to the God and Father of our Lord Jesus Christ, the Father of compassion and the God of all comfort, who comforts us in all our troubles, so that we can comfort those in any trouble with the comfort we ourselves receive from God"* (2 Corinthians 1:3-4 NIV).

"If you live in Me [abide vitally united to Me] and My words remain in you and continue to live in your hearts, ask whatever you will, and it shall be done for you."
John 15:7 (AMP)

CHAPTER 12

Importance of a Second Opinion

I have a great treatment team in Chattanooga. I have tremendous confidence in all members' expertise, care, and experience. It's wonderful to have confidence with our team, but it can also make it difficult to tell them we want another opinion. Once I made the decision to go to MD Anderson, I struggled with telling my oncologist. She had not said anything to cause me to feel hesitant, but I was worried she would not understand why I wanted a second opinion. As usual, I worried without reason. When I told her of my plan to go to MD Anderson, not only did she encourage me but she helped me get all the necessary paperwork sent to MDA. If you decide to pursue another opinion, tell your physician. They can gather and send all the necessary information for you, giving you time to focus on healing.

A dear friend had been treated at MD Anderson for many years and she and her husband helped me maneuver the travel arrangements. I learned that some of the larger research hospitals have hotels nearby that shuttle you to the hospital. Certain airlines will also give discounts when you are flying for medical reasons. Traveling before or during treatment can be challenging, so ask someone to help you plan your trip. Thankfully, my friend's guidance and experience made the process less overwhelming.

Before the appointment I spent countless hours compiling questions regarding triple negative breast cancer. If I was going to be away from Alana for almost a week, travel over 800 miles, and spend the money, I planned to be prepared. Below is the list of questions I took to MD Anderson, in addition to some of the other questions listed in chapter 4. If you feel another opinion will give you comfort, greater understanding of the disease, or help make treatment decisions, I encourage you to seek out another physician experienced with your diagnosis. If you choose to have a second or third opinion, or when talking with anyone on your treatment team, use these questions or adapt them to your specific situation.

- (Name the chemotherapy treatment plan your doctor has prescribed.) Would you recommend the same treatment or something different? Why or why not?
- If your doctor didn't prescribe radiation as part of your treatment plan, ask if they would recommend radiation therapy.
- What is the difference between the MD Anderson treatment chart and the NCCN Guidelines?
- Do I need a PET scan or MUGA scan? If not, what type of scan do you recommend?
- Do you routinely scan? If so, how often?
    - Is it worth being subjected to the radiation?
    - Do you recommend a full-body scan annually after chemo is complete?
- Will you explain the PARP Inhibitor? Would I benefit from it?
- (If you are taking any supplements or vitamins, list them.) Are these beneficial or could they be damaging or related to my diagnosis? Could they counteract my treatment?
- (List any recurring symptoms you have, if any.) Are these symptoms related to the cancer or something different?
- Will you explain blood count results and how they impact my diagnosis?
- Will the chemo affect my heart?
- What are the long-term side effects of the chemo I'm taking?
    - How can I counteract those long-term side effects?
- Do I need genetic testing? Should I take the BART test and BRCA 1 and 2 test?
- Are there any other gene mutation tests I should consider?
- Do you recommend Neulasta or other immune system boosting medication after a chemo treatment?
- When taking Paclitaxel, are the steroids used only to control nausea or do they help make the Taxol more effective? If only for nausea, can we use other medication and decrease the amount of steroids?
- Do chemo side effects normally progress?
- What role does insulin play in my diagnosis?
- Are there ways to normalize insulin levels?
- What are your suggestions for alleviating nausea and mouth sores?
- Why would my cells turn aggressive if they were non-invasive, non-aggressive before?
    - Do you have a theory as to what caused my cancer so I can link it to something tangible?

*****

After recovering from the infection, I had the second A/C treatment. The next day I returned to the chemo room for the Neulasta injection. I had read Claritin D would help, and I was willing to take most anything to lessen the pain. The following week continued as it had after the first treatment, my body hurt to the core of my bones. Every inch ached, it hurt to sit, lie down, or walk.

After that very long week, I began to feel better and continued preparing for the trip to MDA. The University of Texas MD Anderson Cancer Center is one the leading and most respected institutes dedicated solely to cancer research and patient care. I wanted to know the treatment I was receiving in Chattanooga would be the same at a larger research institute. I scheduled an appointment and began the process of gathering all required medical documents to send to Texas. If you elect to visit another facility they will most likely need medical records, the tissue retrieved from surgery, and all the notes and records from each surgery. Thankfully, my oncologist and the staff at Tennessee Oncology helped get all the necessary records to MDA.

While planning the trip to Texas, I was also in the midst of recovering from chemo treatment, another infection, and my recent hair loss. As with most events, there are wonderful memories that come during the most trying of times. One of my sweetest memories happened when I was also exceptionally sick (yes, there were good moments during those days). I had managed to move from the bed to the sofa downstairs and my dad was sitting beside me as I rested. As we talked he brought the conversation to the subject of finances. He said, "Baby, I've decided to sell the '56 Chevy and pay for you to go to MDA." I choked back the tears as I recalled the pride he took in that car and the years he had spent having it restored. But compared to his love for me, the car meant nothing. My heart was filled with gratitude but I asked him to wait before he made that decision. I went on to explain that I was hoping my insurance plan would cover the office visit and I was exploring the most economical way of getting to Houston. He reluctantly agreed to wait but emphasized his desire to help. A few days later, with the help of my friends who frequently visited MDA, I shopped airfare and learned some of the hotels close to the hospital offered medical discounts along with shuttle service to and from the hospital. Thankfully, my dad did not sell the car during that time, but I am forever grateful for this and many other acts of kindness and support during those most difficult days.

*****

During the initial visit at MD Anderson, they ask that you plan to stay at least one week. Alana and I had never been apart for that length of time. September 3, a few days before leaving for Texas, Alana was so upset. She cried as she told me how much she dreaded being away from me for a week. I tried to comfort her with words and prayer but nothing seemed to help. I made every attempt to hide my emotions but I was sick at the thought of leaving. As we continued to talk, I emphasized all the fun she would have staying with our friends while I was gone. She was happy to have sleepovers during the school week, but she wanted our normal life back too.

I dreaded the trip, I dreaded being away from Alana, and I feared the doctors at MD Anderson would find something wrong. "What if surgery had not taken all the cancer?" "What if MDA found something worse than the original diagnosis?" I struggled to control these and many other thoughts.

*****

September 9, making our way to the Atlanta airport proved to be quite the adventure. My brother-in-law and sister-in-law drove Dan, Alana, and me to the airport. The two-hour drive was going smoothly until traffic unexpectedly stopped 45 minutes outside Atlanta. We later learned there had been a high-speed chase and shooting that caused the backup. We missed our flight but a very kind Delta representative was able to get us the last two seats on the 10:00 flight into Houston, which meant that I had more time with Alana. There is always a blessing when you look.

September 2012 I still can't believe all this is happening. I can't believe I'm taking chemo. I'm scared beyond words. I don't want to go to MD Anderson. I don't want to be away from Alana. I'm so worried she will be upset while I'm gone. I hate cancer!

As Alana, my brother-in-law, and sister-in--law started getting ready to head back to Chattanooga, I could tell Alana was anxious. She and I went to the bathroom and she immediately started crying. We held each other as I tried to comfort her, letting her know how quickly the time would go by and how much fun she would have with her friends. I forced smiles rather than the tears I wanted to cry. I kissed her over and over again, wrapping my arms around her so tightly with no desire to let go. My heart was breaking.

When it was time for them to leave, we all walked to the parking garage entrance where we hugged and kissed again. I stood motionless and silent as I watched them walk away. Alana turned around a few times to look back and wave. I held my tears until she was out of sight.

As Dan and I walked back inside, the terminal felt suffocating. I needed to be outside. We found a bench at the drop-off area and the uncontrollable tears came. That night outside of the Atlanta airport I threw myself a pity party. I missed Alana terribly, I felt sorry for myself because of the diagnosis, I felt sorry for myself because of the treatment. I also felt sorry for myself because I knew I wasn't holding every thought captive and was allowing Satan to control me with fear. Looking down at my watch I realized it was the time I would normally be making Alana's lunch for the next school day. I longed to be home with our normal routine rather than getting ready to board a flight to an institute that may tell me worse news about my condition. There are no words to describe the emotional agony this diagnosis can bring.

We sat outside the airport for nearly two hours, Dan sitting patiently by my side as I cried out my frustrations. When I finally gained some composure, I focused my thoughts on prayer. I asked Jesus over and over, "Please don't take me from her. Please don't make me leave her." My eyes were lifted up toward heaven, my lips quietly pleading for continued life. In that moment I heard God speak directly into my heart: *"I'm not."* The words were so clear that at first I was taken aback. Did I really just hear that? Did I just feel that? This was the first time in my life I'd felt deep in my soul that I heard the voice of God. Not all of my fear was eliminated, but there was an all-consuming peace in that moment that everything was going to be okay.

September 11, 2012, Dan and I walked through the massive MD Anderson campus. I was filled with anxiety but, again, God was good and granted peace. I was prepared to meet this well-known triple negative specialist. I had 25 questions ready to go. I did not intend to go through all I had to get here and not be prepared.

During the appointment she thoroughly went over my pathology report, treatment plan, and statistical chance of recurrence. She explained they would offer the same treatment plan I was receiving with the exception of a minor brand difference with one of the drugs. She said, as I already knew, triple negative is not estrogen, progesterone, or HER2 driven. She went on to explain there could be a genetic component, possibly BRCA 1, BRCA 2, or BART but the statistical probability was low. We discussed the possibility of additional genetic testing once I returned to Chattanooga. We agreed genetic testing can cause fear, but I wanted to know the statistical possibility of passing a gene mutation to my daughter and possibly her children. See chapter 19 for additional information regarding genetic testing.

Because MD Anderson's diagnosis and treatment plan was almost exactly the same as my current plan, I only needed the one appointment and to return the following day for copies of my medical reports. The second day there I visited the "barber shop." MDA provides each patient one free wig, so I chose long brown hair very similar to my natural hair. If you go to another facility for a second opinion, always look into their resources. It was a nice treat to get a new (and free) wig.

I was ready to go home but when I called to change our flights the additional charge was considerably more if we traveled on Wednesday. If we waited until Thursday and flew out of another airport the flight change fee was much less. Although I desperately wanted to go home, I decided to make the most of our time there. Again, if we can't change our circumstances we must change our thoughts. The following day, Wednesday, Dan and I rented a car and drove to Galveston beach. We enjoyed walking along the beach and having pizza by the shore. It was a wonderful day, but I couldn't wait to be home with Alana.

I am continually amazed how God provides opportunities to practice compassion while also causing us to focus less on ourselves. The second morning as we boarded the shuttle a young child and her mother were among our group of passengers. The child looked to be around Alana's age. She was bald and her skin, a shade of blue/gray, was covered in large, raised lesions. I could not imagine what this child had endured in her short life. My heart ached as I fought back tears. I was filled with compassion while also consumed with gratitude for my daughter's health. I prayed for her then and continue to pray each time I think of this precious little girl.

Our cancer journey will continue to be filled with moments like this one—moments where we experience the odd combination of gratitude and grief. As contradictory as it sounds, these two emotions frequently mix. There will be moments along this journey when you feel completely worn down from grieving your condition and yet you are filled with gratitude for the small blessings of life, whether that is the health of your family or simply being able to spend a night in with friends. Though these emotions strongly combat each other, try your best to make gratitude shine brighter. A spirit of gratefulness really can uplift and brighten those bad days.

"People always ask me how long it takes to do my hair. I don't know, I'm never there."
Dolly Parton

CHAPTER 13

How to Wear a Wig…
On a Rollercoaster

You may have read about the day my hair began its departure in chapter 11, but losing our hair is such an important part of the cancer journey that I've also included this event in the wig chapter. Alana was eight years old and had finished second grade a couple weeks before my cancer diagnosis.It was now August and time to register for third grade. So much had happened and much more lie ahead but that morning we were excited to register and meet her teachers. As we were getting ready to go, I brushed through my hair and quickly realized large chunks of hair were on my brush. Whenever you start chemo they tell you this will eventually happen, but many people, myself included, have a small voice in the back of their mind saying they might be the one-in-a-million exception. Turns out, I wasn't the exception. I was two weeks past my first treatment and already losing my hair. I sat on the edge of the tub and cried. I had been warned but nothing can prepare us ladies for the day when we wake with a head full of hair and realize we will be bald within days.

I clutched my hair in one hand and called Dan with the other. Through tears I told him my hair had started falling out. He tried to console me, telling me it didn't matter if I lost my hair. Thinking back to that conversation, I am reminded of how incredibly lucky I am to have a husband who doesn't care if his wife is bald. Though miniscule in the big picture, in the moment, for me, this was a huge ordeal. I had long brown hair before starting chemo, and here it was in my hands, each strand slowly abandoning ship.

After I regained my composure, I explained to Alana that my hair had started coming out and I would need to wear a hat to registration. She knew this was going to happen and didn't seem too concerned. A few minutes later my precious daughter emerged from her room wearing a hat. We proudly rocked those hats for third grade registration.

Shortly after my hair started coming out, I had eleven inches cut off and donated. I was careful after the haircut to preserve as much of my hair as possible so Alana could shave it off. I wouldn't brush or comb through it and I wore a ball cap most of the time. I wanted the moment my head was shaved to be a special memory for Alana to recall in the midst of the sickness and trials ahead. So we waited until I mustered up enough strength and then spent an afternoon playing salon.

The day Alana shaved my head was a beautiful, clear August day. We set up our salon on the back deck complete with spray bottle, spray conditioner, combs, and salon scissors to make it official. I put on my vampire cape (part of a Halloween costume, in case you wondered why I had vampire attire). The vampire cape served as the perfect substitute for a salon cape. I sat in the chair ready for my new look. Alana could cut my hair anyway she wanted. We laughed, talked, and took funny pictures as she snipped along. We shared a wonderful, cheerful afternoon. There were no tears! Our deck is private, so we were able to keep this moment just between the two of us. Allowing Alana to shave my head was one way of taking a negative situation and turning it into a fun day we would happily remember. After all, it's not every day that a child gets to cut and shave their mom's hair!

*****

Prior to starting chemotherapy, I recommend finding at least one wig, a fitted scarf to sleep in, a few scarves to wear over your head, and a ball cap with or without attached hair (the hair is sewn into the cap giving it a very realistic look). I wish I had taken more time to shop for a wig prior to losing my hair but I did not. I knew I did not want my appearance to change drastically and I had found a wig I liked but had no idea how to wear or care for the hair. I wore ball caps frequently but wigs, extensions, and scarves were all foreign. I have so much respect for women who choose not to wear any type of head covering but I was not one of them.

I had gone to look at wigs before beginning chemo but assumed there would be more time to shop before my hair came out. I was wrong again. A couple weeks after my first chemo treatment, as I lay on the couch recovering from an infection, my cousin came over for a visit. While we talked she handed me a box. I cried when I opened the box and saw the wig I had tried on during my only visit to a wig salon. She had gone to the salon and found the wig I liked then told her siblings and family what she planned to do. They all pitched in and bought my first new wig. I held the beautiful pieces of hair, relieved to know I would now have hair once I was recovered enough to venture out. Her thoughtfulness and generosity could not have come at a better time.

With practice and help from Gerri, at The Wig Palace, I learned to be quick and proficient with my wig. No one ever knew I was wearing a wig unless I chose to tell them. I was in a wedding shortly after finishing chemo when my friend and I went to a salon for makeup. While there she also had her hair styled. The hairdresser asked if I wanted to have my hair styled in an up-do. She had no idea I was wearing a wig, she thought I was joking when I explained my "hair." She had all the other hairdressers look at my hair. I finally pulled up the edges to prove the hair was not natural.

Wigs can be such an important resource and a way to bring back a sense of normalcy to our daily lives. Honestly, my natural hair never looked as good as my wigs. Another bonus is the time saved. You can have fabulous, celebrity-style hair in less than two minutes. What a bonus! Whether you purchase the same style you had before chemo or try something that has always piqued your interest, have fun with this temporary phase in your life.

If you don't immediately embrace your new hair (wig), understand this is normal too. If you're like me, I had no idea what to expect. Since my diagnosis, I have met women who choose to wear wigs for many different reasons, but each will most likely admit it took time to get accustomed to the way they feel on your head. Some describe them as heavy or hot. I did not experience either. Once I found the first wig that fit and looked good, I considered it my hair. I did all activities including hiking and working out with my hair. I would clip it into an up-do, a pony tail, or any other style. Don't be afraid to try different styles with your new hair!

A few weeks after finishing chemo, my family and I went to Disney World with friends. As you may know, Disney World has roller coasters and many other wind-blowing rides. Anyone who has ever worn a wig will tell you one of the greatest fears is that the wind will blow the wig right off your head. This is not a vision most want to imagine. I was determined to ride every coaster with Alana AND keep my hair attached.

Admittedly, I did not know how I would accomplish this goal. As we stood in line for the first roller coaster, I prayed. God instructs us to pray about everything, so I prayed my hair would stay on my head. As the coaster approached, I decided I would keep one hand in front of Alana and the other firmly placed on top of my head. It was February and I was sweating. I held my breath as the coaster started.

I'm happy (and grateful) to report my hair stayed in place. As we exited and looked for our picture on the display, we laughed at the sight of my hand on top of my head in every picture. The next day my friend had the brilliant idea that I should wear her jacket with an attached hood. Once seated on the ride, I would tie the hood as tight as possible under my chin. Again, I would keep my hand in front of Alana but I now had my other free to hold the bar. And that, my friends, is how you wear a wig and ride a roller coaster.

*****

I get more questions about hair than I do the surgeries. Hair, or more importantly the lack of, is a vital part of the treatment and recovery process. I've been asked many times, "How long does it take before your hair starts to fall out?" For me, it started on day fourteen after my first treatment. The next question is, "How long before it starts to come back?" Unfortunately, there isn't an exact timeline. I know some whose hair came back earlier and others who took much longer, but here is the path my hair followed. Two months and two weeks post-chemo my hair started to grow but it didn't feel like hair. If you have ever held a baby chick and felt their fur, that was the texture. Prior to treatment my hair was fine but this new "fuzz" went far beyond fine and it was not coming back consistently. I had about an inch of hair right above both ears and along my neck line. The remaining part of my head was covered with about a quarter inch of this new fuzz (it really didn't qualify to be called hair).

July 2013, six months past my last chemo treatment, I had enough growth that it required my first shampoo and condition. I did not consider giving up my wigs or ball cap (with attached hair), but my hair was growing. A month later, one year after losing my hair, it was growing back curly. I had more hair in the back along my neckline and above my ear than I did on top. The color was very similar to the color before chemo. At least I think it was the same, I hadn't really seen my natural color (except the roots) in years. As most, I wanted a different hair color than the one God chose for me. Most of us Southern girls like blonde, but not me. I wanted dark hair. Yet, God chose to make me (almost) blonde twice, once at birth and then after chemo.

October 2013, nine months past the last chemo treatment, I had a full blown mullet. To all the ladies out there who can sport this look, rock on! Unfortunately, I was not in the group. This style was not my first choice but was better than bald... maybe. The hair along my neckline was blonde and curly but the top sections still weren't coming in as consistently as the back. I continued to wear my wig but I would exercise with only a ball cap. My blonde curls peeked out the back of the cap just enough to give the illusion of "normal" hair. The following month I had my first haircut since losing all my hair.

WIG DO'S AND DON'TS

I knew absolutely nothing about wigs, how to wear them, or where to find different styles and colors. So, I did my homework. I researched all things hair and found an excellent resource in my hometown. If you live anywhere close to the Southeast, I highly recommend visiting The Wig Palace. I found this treasure in the heart of Chattanooga, TN. The owner, Gerri, had been a hairdresser for over 20 years when she bought the salon. She taught me how to wear, style, clean, and condition my new hair. I enjoyed my wigs and continued to wear them long after my hair came back. Along the way, and with Gerri's help, I learned a few tips:

- Most of us start out thinking we want human hair. I assumed this would be the best option, however, I quickly learned synthetic wigs look just as realistic, are cheaper, and far easier to maintain.
- Ask if your healthcare policy will cover the cost of a wig. If so, your oncologist can write the prescription. My insurance did not cover the cost but it's always best to ask.
- Never put heat on your wig. Leave this to the professionals.
- Be careful taking food out of the oven. The heat can actually cause your wig to fray, especially if you have bangs.
- You never want your hair to scream wig! To avoid this common mistake, I recommend replacing the wig once the ends start to look frayed. Nothing

screams wig like stiff, ratty strands!

- I stored my wigs on wig stands and wig heads. Be careful with the Styrofoam heads as they can stretch a wig.
- I kept my wigs on a shelf in my closet. Alana knew her friends should not go into my closet, but my biggest concern was that one of her friends would open the door and find two or three faceless heads with long brown hair staring back at her! For most eight-year-olds this sight would add years to their future therapy sessions.
- One of the biggest mistakes I made early on was washing my wig too often. Don't wash your wig more than every 6-8 weeks unless you sweat a lot or your wig needs to be conditioned. Some say the wig makes their head sweat but I did not have this problem. I hiked, worked out, and did most all activities wearing my wig.
- Use only wig shampoo and conditioner to clean your wig. Follow the instructions and add a small amount of shampoo to the sink or a bowl of cold water, move the wig around in the water, then condition as directed. I would hang my wig inside-out to dry. Warning: The wig will look like a "ratty" wet animal hanging from your shower. The first time I cleaned my wig I thought I had destroyed it. I was so upset. I was going on a field trip with my daughter's third grade class the following morning and feared I had nothing to wear... on my head.
- If possible, have more than one wig. After the field trip scare I always had at least a couple hair choices. One of my friends has a short wig for warm days and a slightly longer wig for more dress up occasions.
- Have fun with colors and styles. Use this as an opportunity to try new looks. I stayed in the brown and auburn colors, but it was fun to explore platinum blonde and other fun colors.
- I would place a napkin under my wig, between my head and the wig.
- Always use a wig brush because other brushes can damage the hair.

TIPS FOR HAIR EXTENSIONS

When your hair starts coming in, hair extensions are a great way to add fullness as it grows back. I explored tape-in extensions, sew extensions, and beaded but did not choose any of these options because I feared they would damage my newly growing hair. I chose to use clip-in hair extensions; these were my first experience with clip-in hair. I used the extensions when I wanted my hair to appear thicker, especially along the base close to my neck. Clip-in extensions give the same fullness as the taped and glued variety, especially along the bottom section of your hair. The biggest drawback is learning how to hide the clips. Gerri, again, taught me the correct way to place the clips. After much trial and error, I learned to pull part of my hair onto the top of my head, leaving the middle section and below to attach the clip. With the crown part of my hair pulled up, I then took a one-inch section of hair and lightly backcombed and sprayed that small piece, being careful not to overspray. Once the hair was backcombed (formerly known as teasing) and sprayed, I clipped the extension to that section of hair. Once you have as many extensions in place as you want, take the hair that was pulled on top of your head and let it fall. This hair will camouflage the clips.

I purchased the packet of extensions but after experimenting chose to use only the side pieces. Extensions are a wonderful option for those whose hair did not return evenly distributed but, like most new styles, they require practice and patience. If you don't like them immediately, keep trying or find a stylist to help. If you choose to have a stylist place your extensions, they will work with you and teach you how to clean and wear your new hair. If you choose the clip-in variety, I recommend watching YouTube. There are some excellent videos that show how to place the hair for the best results.

HAIR TOPPERS, BANGS, AND FILLERS

When hair starts to return it's generally thinner in the front along the hair line. I've always liked wearing my hair in a ponytail or bun but after chemo my hair was still thin and my scalp would show. While exploring in Ulta and Sally Beauty Supply, I came across hair building fibers made by Toppik, Viviscal, and Ion. These miraculous hair fibers fill in thinning areas but were especially helpful for the section above my bangs. I bought a small container and followed the instructions, shaking the fibers onto the thinner areas. Immediately my hair looked thicker and fuller. I loved the results! I bought the Toppik spray to hold the fibers in place but I found hairspray works just as well. Once in place, I would check my face to be certain none of the fibers fell from the hair. If so, simply wipe them off with a cloth or make up brush.

I found these fibers stay in place through rain, sweat, and wind. The only time they came off unwanted was on my pillow. I woke one morning to find two strange dark spots on my white pillow. To remedy this, each evening before going to bed I would quickly run my fingers through the covered area. The fibers fall into the sink and not on the pillow, problem solved. I really enjoyed this product when wearing my favorite up-do—the messy bun.

I also went to a local salon to investigate what is known as "halo hair." This is hair sewn onto a thin "fish line" type material. The hair was great but very thick and expensive (for my budget). I didn't want my look to change so drastically, taking my hair from average fullness to very thick.

As I continued looking, I found another halo-type hair piece at Sally's Beauty Supply for a fraction of the cost. The hair is thinner but comes two in a pack. I took one of the pieces of hair to Gerri at the Wig Palace. She cut the hair to blend beautifully with my natural hair. This hair doesn't solve the thinning crown area but it's an excellent option if you want thicker, longer looking hair. The only problem I found is completely concealing the thin fish line. To remedy this, spray paint the clear colored line brown or a shade close to your hair color. Wearing a head band would also conceal the line in the places where hair doesn't completely cover.

I have purchased several types of clip-in bangs but each was too thick. Some looked as though I had a small animal clipped onto my forehead—not my ideal look. I found one possible option at Sally's Beauty Supply. Hair2wear makes clip-in bangs that are thinner and more natural looking. The clips can be used to fill in areas along the crown or cut to fill in thinning bangs. The problem is concealing the clips. It's difficult to conceal clips in an area where the hair is already thin. With practice and enough hair the clips can hide under small sections of hair, but beware, if someone much taller stands beside you and inspects your scalp your clips might be visible.

My hair eventually came back curlier, fuller, and thicker than ever before but I continue to explore extensions, especially for the crown and bangs. However, I have yet to find anything natural looking and affordable. Several salons have great options for extensions but most cater to making the hair longer or fuller along the baseline. Stay tuned and continue to check the website for possible solutions.

"Keep your face always toward the sunshine –
and shadows will fall behind you."
Walt Whitman

CHAPTER 14

Appearances Can Be Deceiving If You Try Hard Enough

Along with the physical side effects of a cancer diagnosis (sickness, nausea, mouth/throat sores, etc.), your outward appearance can also be affected. We've covered the hair (pun intended), but there are other ways your appearance can be impacted. There will be times when you catch a glimpse of your reflection and it completely blindsides you. This happened to me in January 2013, shortly before my last chemo treatment. Alana and I were dancing in the kitchen to one of our favorite songs, "You Make Me Smile," when I caught a glimpse of my reflection in the window and burst into tears. In that short moment, it was overwhelming. I was overcome with my love for Alana and overwhelmed that I really was that lady with the scarf. I began to cry as we danced. Dan then joined us and we all held each other and danced. My husband gently said, "It's a temporary look for a permanent fix." As you go through this chapter with tips on normalizing your appearance through and after chemo, I hope you remember this is a temporary issue on the road to recovery or remission.

By the end of treatment my eyebrows and eyelashes were scarce but still hanging on. A couple weeks post-treatment, they were gone. I started practicing make-up tricks that gave the appearance of eyebrows and eyelashes. Thanks to chemo, I was bald, void of eyebrows and eyelashes with ghostly pale grayish toned skin (not my most attractive stage in life). That was one way of looking at my situation but there was always another perspective. My hair was fabulous, better than my long-gone "real" hair, I was thinner than I'd been in a while, and I could always spray tan (I didn't but it was an option).

Proverbs 31 reminds us "beauty is fleeting" but... we still want to hang on to it as long as possible. Here are a few of the tricks I explored during this appearance challenging time.

ADDING EYEBROWS AND EYELASHES:

Each morning I would take a dark brown eyebrow pencil and color in where my eyebrows once were. I would then take a lighter brown eyebrow pencil and go over that same line. Using two colors helped give them a more natural look. I would then take an eyebrow brush and brush in an upward motion so the brows would not have a sharp drawn on look (this look never worked on me). If needed, I would then take a cotton swab and shape the brows into their natural arch while gently removing any thicker lines from the pencil. This method worked wonders for the brows.

Almost as quickly as the eyebrows and eyelashes disappeared, they began to grow back. They started as tiny pieces of fuzz but quickly grew back slightly thicker than before treatment. My hair did not respond as quickly.

SKIN AND NAIL CONCERNS:

In August 2013, the last remaining visible signs of chemo were my hair (lack of) and nails. I did not lose any of my fingernails or toenails, but many people do experience the nail completely detaching and coming off. One of my friends had to have two fingernails removed during chemo treatment. She wore Band-Aids to cover the nail loss. All of my fingernails turned a chalky shade of gray but did not detach. They were never sore or painful, although this is somewhat common. The nail bed on each of my big toes turned the same chalky white/gray color but did not come off. I did not wear nail polish often before treatment and chose not to wear it during treatment.

I took a B complex vitamin to help with the nail loss but recommend doing your homework before taking these supplements. Some forms of B supplements are natural and some are synthetic. If you are considering vitamins, supplements, or any holistic supplementation, we have excellent resources in the Chattanooga area. The team at Nutrition World is extremely knowledgeable and can help with any nutrition or dietary needs. In the Hixson area, The Family Herb Shop carries many supplements, vitamins, and herbal solutions. Both shops are knowledgeable, affordable, compassionate, and well stocked for all your nutritional needs. See chapter 15 for additional nutrition information. Most importantly, talk with your doctor before taking any vitamin or supplement. Some supplements can interfere with chemotherapy.

Prior to chemo, my complexion was normal to oily. However, during treatment my skin was extremely dry. I switched to skin care for dry skin and would often use organic coconut oil before going to bed. The coconut oil helped and was much more affordable than some skin care products.

Your oncologist will most likely recommend avoiding sun exposure during chemo. I am a firm believer in the importance of natural Vitamin D from the sun but during treatment I used a lot of sunscreen. Chemotherapy can make your skin hyper-sensitive to the sun. I sat outside no more than 10 minutes without sunscreen once and was close to sunburnt. Lather on the sunscreen!

CLOTHING HACKS:

As with any major change to your appearance, people have a natural curiosity about the part of your body that has been transformed. Whether you've had reconstruction or not, people know there is something different lurking beneath the fibers of your clothing and they can't help but look. When you have had breast cancer, people have a tendency to try to steal peeks at your chest, especially when they are seeing you for the first time since surgery. Just for the record, we know what you are doing. If we look away for a second, the glance goes to our chest. Understandable (somewhat) but keep the glances to a minimum or (better) not at all.

If you're under construction (AKA reconstruction) or chose not to have reconstruction there are a few tips that can help camouflage that now sacred part of your body until you become comfortable returning to your former wardrobe. Wearing stripes or printed tops is helpful as patterns conceal more than solids. I've also experimented with and heard many women talk about the success of layering clothing. If you elected not to reconstruct, wearing a padded sports bra at the gym or underneath any clothing can give the illusion of breasts. Prosthetics and knitted knockers (yep, that's the name) offer removable breasts. If you are under construction and don't want to appear larger than before surgery, wear a tight sports bra. If that doesn't work, add another sports bra, sometimes two will give the desired coverage better than one. Larger, thick cardigans provide good coverage if weather allows. Play around with necklines as well. Certain necklines may reveal too much too soon or not enough depending on your desired appearance. It's all trial and error with this new body, but view this as a time to branch out with your style and enjoy clothing your new, beautiful body.

"If you can't fly then run, if you can't run then walk, if you can't walk then crawl, but whatever you do you have to keep moving forward."
Martin Luther King, Jr.

CHAPTER 15

Nutrition During and After Treatment

I assumed I would lose weight during chemo treatments. As with most assumptions, I was wrong. In fact, one of the more common misconceptions about chemotherapy is that you'll lose a lot of weight. The truth is some people actually gain weight during chemo. Whether you gain or lose, this is certainly not the time to diet.

Chemo can also bring appetite changes, making some foods, even your favorites, completely unappealing. I've always enjoyed a variety of foods, primarily healthier choices, but during the more severe side effects I wanted only potatoes and saltine crackers. I rarely eat either, but when the nausea was at its worst saltine crackers were my go-to. Once the nausea began to subside, potatoes were all I craved. Potatoes in any form were appealing—mashed, baked, in soup, or alone, it didn't matter. Thankfully, my mom, sister, and niece kept the potatoes coming.

Once diagnosed you will be given a notebook filled with excellent nutrition information. If you don't have the time or energy to read all the information, below are highlights from a registered dietician who works with oncology nutrition.

- Stay hydrated. Hydration helps flush out all those extra chemicals left in the blood stream from chemo. Staying hydrated helps everything in the body work better. Try to drink a lot of water, but drink alternatives if you develop an aversion to water or struggle with a metallic taste. I generally prefer water but lemonade became my temporary favorite. Try to stay away from sugary fluids like soda.

- Don't wait too long between meals and don't eat too much during a meal. The oncology nutritionist used this analogy: if you were going to drive from Tennessee to California you couldn't get all your gas in just one stop, you would have to make many stops along the way. Don't eat one huge meal then nothing the rest of the day. Keep something on your stomach to help combat nausea.

- Try to have a form of protein at every meal.
- If you are worried about organic versus non-organic, follow the "dirty dozen" list. It can be expensive to buy only organic, but some fruits and veggies are more susceptible to pesticides than others.
- I've always believed in the 80/20 system—80% of our meals we try to eat clean and healthy but the other 20% is probably made up of chips and some form of sugar. Alana and I came up with this example: we have two armies in our bodies – the good and the bad. Who do you want to feed? It's okay to feed the bad army occasionally, but feed the good army more often. It's a great rule before and after you finish treatment, but I couldn't follow it during treatment. I became the queen of carbs—potatoes, potatoes, potatoes.
- Obey your "off limits" food rules for chemo—sushi, raw and undercooked meat, buffets, Caesar salad, etc. Your immune system will be compromised. Be sure to get this list from your oncologist or nutritionist.
- To keep side effects at bay during chemotherapy, eat smaller meals more frequently throughout the day.
- When you are sick, eat when you can and what you can.
- It's okay to drink your nutrients if that's all you can keep down.

DURING TREATMENT

During treatment there are a number of side effects you may experience that impact appetite and diet. Luckily, there are certain things you can do to combat these – sometimes extremely unpleasant and gross – side effects[8].

Diarrhea
- Drink plenty of liquids, preferably non-fizzy, at room temperature
- Eat 5-6 smaller meals instead of 3 big meals
- Eat low fiber foods

Dry mouth
- Sip on water throughout the day to keep your mouth moistened
- Drink very sweet or very tart drinks like lemonade to produce saliva
  - Pro Tip: Do not drink these kinds of liquids if you have mouth sores as they might make them worse
- Chew gum, suck on hard candy or ice chips
- Eat easy-to-swallow foods or foods that have been softened

Nausea
- Eat food that is easy on the stomach, not spicy meals
- Eat smaller meals more frequently – don't skip meals!

- Sip small amounts of liquid throughout the day to keep something on your stomach
- Eat foods that appeal to you
  - Pro Tip: Try to stay away from your favorite foods when nauseated so you don't associate them with being sick. I learned the hard way that chemo and salmon was not a good combination.

Sore mouth/throat
- Eat soft food that is easy to swallow – cook food until it is tender
- Drink liquids through a straw
- Avoid hot food and drinks – eat food and drink liquids that are either cold or room temperature
- Suck on ice chips
- Avoid foods that may hurt your mouth/throat, especially foods that are sour, spicy, salty, or sharp

Sickness/vomiting
- Drink clear liquids until you can keep solids down
- Slowly add full liquids and neutral foods back into your diet
- Eat small meals more frequently
- The saltine crackers your grandma gave you as a child could be helpful too

Constipation
- Drink lots of liquids, preferably hot liquids and room temperature fluids
- Eat high-fiber foods (Fiber One Cereal can be helpful)
- Talk with your doctor before taking laxatives or other constipation medicine
- Stay active—daily activity can help relieve this side effect

*Most importantly, contact your doctor when experiencing consistent side effects. He or she can't help you if they don't know.

PREVENTION

We all know there is no magic pill that can cure or prevent all cancer (unfortunately), but there are certain foods that contain nutrients your body needs to fight against harmful enemy cells. There have been many studies that show a higher body mass index (BMI) increases your risk for cancer. Though this is not a direct, finger-pointing correlation (because cancer is still a very unpredictable and mysterious beast), an argument can be made for the benefits of a balanced lifestyle. The following are a few ways medical professionals suggest for a more health-conscious anti-cancer diet[9].

- Diets that are primarily plant-based (i.e. fruits and vegetables) have high nutrient counts and low calorie counts, which help in maintaining a lower body weight. Experts actually say that most of our plates should be plant-based with less processed food and food that is high in fat—especially red meat. My deepest apologies to all you dedicated carnivores out there.

- Going through cancer treatments greatly increases your risk of infection because treatment can weaken your immune system. Because your body is vulnerable, most members of your treatment team will tell you not to consume raw or undercooked meat, such as sushi or very pink steak. You should also be very cautious when handling raw meat – if you handle it at all – and always scrub your raw fruits and vegetables thoroughly before eating.

- Your doctor may also suggest you cut down or eliminate alcohol during treatment. Several studies have been conducted that show a correlation between breast cancer and alcohol. Talk with your doctor about alcohol. Be honest about frequency and amounts—yes, there is a size difference between a wine glass and a fish bowl.

NUTRITION SITES

There are many great resources regarding nutrition during and after chemo. I gained a lot of useful tips from *"The Whole-Food Guide for Breast Cancer Survivors: A Nutritional Approach to Preventing Recurrence"* by Edward Bauman. This book provides excellent nutritional and lifestyle information whether you're in treatment, have completed treatment, or are simply trying to enjoy a healthier plate. The following are also nutrition resource sites you can visit for more information:

- **The American Cancer Society** *(cancer.org)* – Click on the "Stay Healthy" tab for helpful tools, nutrition charts, and up-to-date articles regarding the latest cancer-related research.

- **American Institute of Cancer** *(aicr.org)* – This site contains a lot of information about preventative cancer nutrition, as well as many yummy recipes you can try post-treatment to maintain a healthy, balanced diet.

- **Abbott Nutrition** *(abbottnutrition.com)* – To easily find what you're looking for on this site, search for "Adult Therapeutic Nutrition"-"Condition Driven"-"Oncology." There you will find professional information about meeting your nutritional needs during treatment.

- **Fruits & Veggies More Matters** *(fruitsandveggiesmorematters.org)* – Working in collaboration with the CDC, this organization has tons of recipes, tips, and information on how to incorporate more fruits and vegetables into your daily diet.

"Mama Llama's always near even if she's not right here."
Anna Dewdney, Llama Llama Red Pajama

CHAPTER 16

A Little Motivation from One Mom to Another

I am not claiming expertise nor do I claim to have all the answers on how to parent during chemo; I just have a lot of practice. Most of the women I have interviewed and talked with tell me their children are their greatest concern. Our kids are our first thought when we hear, "You have cancer," and they are our greatest motivation during treatments. Whatever our parenting norms, they will be different during cancer treatment. I wanted desperately for Alana's life to continue as close to normal as possible but I also knew we would all have to adjust to our new normal. As much as you may want your usual routine to continue, try to accept the temporary changes and look for the positives they will bring.

Dan, Alana, and I vowed from the beginning we would tackle this illness as a family. I feel strongly that being open and honest, using age appropriate terminology with Alana, helped reduce her fears. I answered any question she had about the cancer, treatment, or how I felt as honestly as possible. We also consistently read scripture to reinforce our belief in God's healing power.

One of my fondest memories is of Alana playing the violin for me. When I was so sick I could only move from the bed to the sofa, she would place cold washcloths on my head between songs. As much as I hated being sick I knew in my heart Alana was learning a new level of compassion. When you are feeling your worst and know you're not at your parenting best, try to look at the situation through even the slightest positive lens. Asking your child to help when you are sick makes them a part of your healing process – they are not a bystander but a participant with your care. When she/he can only watch helplessly they can feel out of control, bringing on more fear. Asking for help also gives them an opportunity to experience a greater level of compassion and empathy than most "normal" life circumstances provide.

Maintaining a balance between your child participating in your care and continuing their usual fun activities, sports, etc. can be a struggle, but incorporating both will give your child an increased sense of compassion while they also enjoy more time than usual with their friends and family. This balance between normalcy and care participation will look different depending on the age of your child or children.

Like most moms, my daughter has been the center of my world since the day she was born. Other than my relationship with God, she is my purpose and greatest joy in life. I went from full-time to very part-time (aka I rarely worked) immediately after we had Alana. Once she started school I was blessed to have the flexibility to work during her school hours. We have been very fortunate to have most of our free time together and with family and friends. Needless to say, we were about to enter a different stage.

Once we had all worked through the initial shock of learning I had cancer, we knew our everyday lifestyle would change but we weren't sure what this new temporary normal would look like. I was diagnosed in June, a time when we would normally be hiking, kayaking, swimming, and all the other usual summer activities but we knew this summer would be different. As much as I wanted to be the one taking Alana on all our adventures, I knew this would not always be possible. Thankfully, we have the most amazing people in our life.

I am forever indebted to my closest friends who made certain Alana's life continued as normal as possible. She went on many fun adventures and spent endless hours with friends that love her dearly. The week following each A/C treatment I was very sick. During most of these days after treatment, one of my friends would pick up Alana and she would spend the day with them and their children. She saw movies, went swimming, hiking, and had more play dates than I can count. Each evening during our nightly devotion, she would enthusiastically tell me about her day.

Peppered throughout these days when I was so sick was the balancing act I spoke of. Dan would leave early for work and Alana would be "in charge" of my care. She would bring crackers, soup, potatoes, or anything I needed. I was well taken care of by my amazing eight year old! We would lie in bed and watch television or simply talk, later she would head out for another fun filled day. Knowing she was having fun gave me more joy than these incredible women will ever know.

I encourage you to lean on others for support while you are recovering from surgeries and/or treatment. Yes, you want to be the one taking your daughter to practice or your son to his big game, but there will be days when it will be physically impossible. Don't attempt to do everything or be afraid to ask for help from friends or family. Lean on people who love you and your children, give them this time to enjoy each other and strengthen their bond with your child.

Keeping time in perspective also helped during the days and weeks I was sick. I would constantly remind myself this period of sickness is short compared to the rest of my life. In the wise words of my husband, "This is a temporary time for a permanent fix." Remember parents: if your life was spread out on a ruler, this time period would only take up a small portion along the entire stretch of life. When you feel your worst, when your spirits are low, try to remember YOU WILL FEEL BETTER. Yes, this too shall pass.

*****

While going through chemotherapy your immune system is compromised. Oncologists advise us to stay away from schools or any gathering that could potentially be a germ playground. I followed the majority of recommendations from my doctors (no sushi, food bars, Caesar salad, etc.) but not this one. I had been homeroom mom since Alana started kindergarten and cancer was not going to stop me this year. Right or wrong (in hindsight – it was wrong), I went to every function, every performance, and all events both in and out of the classroom. I continued my weekly volunteer time except the weeks I was too sick to go. Let me emphasize, I would not recommend anyone else do this – I was putting myself in a situation to potentially get very sick. I wanted so desperately for Alana's school days to be normal that I risked further illness. I am in no way promoting my choices. In hindsight, they were not the best.

*****

Don't be surprised if something completely pierces your heart when you least expect it, even years past your diagnosis. January 2014, it had been over two years since learning I had cancer but those past raw emotions still showed up without warning. One evening as Alana and I were looking through our books we noticed a book she loved when she was younger. We were playing and being silly so she sat on my lap and asked me to read the book as I did when she was little. When I came to the page where the Mama Llama was calming her upset child, I read, "Mama Llama's always near even if she's not right here" (Dewdney, 2005). The words brought unexpected tears. They express what most moms feel in any situation, but maybe even more so when face-to-face with cancer. Moms are always near, whether we are in the next room or miles away.

Parenting during recovery, chemo, radiation, reconstruction, etc. is tough. Juggling the emotions cancer brings is even more difficult. While you are traveling over this rocky terrain of cancer remember your child is traveling with you. Tell them what is going on, let them know what to expect, allow them to take care of you, and, when you are sick, send them for fun adventures with those who love them too.

This chapter is dedicated to my closest friends. The term "friend" does not adequately describe our relationship. We are family. We've been through so many of life's difficulties together, far too many to name. These ladies know who they are. I am forever grateful for the peace they gave me during the most difficult time of my life. Knowing my daughter was with any one of them gave me joy during the darkest moments. I thank God for the laughter, tears, and all the wonderful stories we share. As we grow older we will have a lifetime of adventures to recall, some with laughter, maybe a little crying, and, if we're lucky, even a little embarrassment.

*****

And for any children who may be struggling with fear or uncertainty for a mother with cancer, my daughter Alana has a word of encouragement for you:

"Hi, this is Alana. My mom was diagnosed with breast cancer when I was eight years old. When I first found out, I was so scared, this was one of my worst memories in my life. I just want to tell you to hold on to God's promises and lean on Him when you are worried. One thing that helped me when I was scared was to sit down and talk to God. I prayed to Him every day and still do."

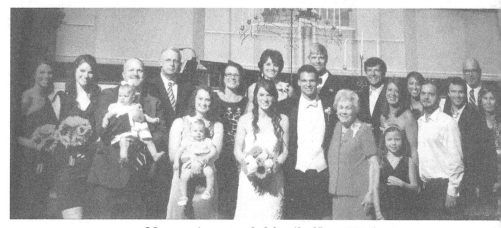

My amazing extended family (June 2013)

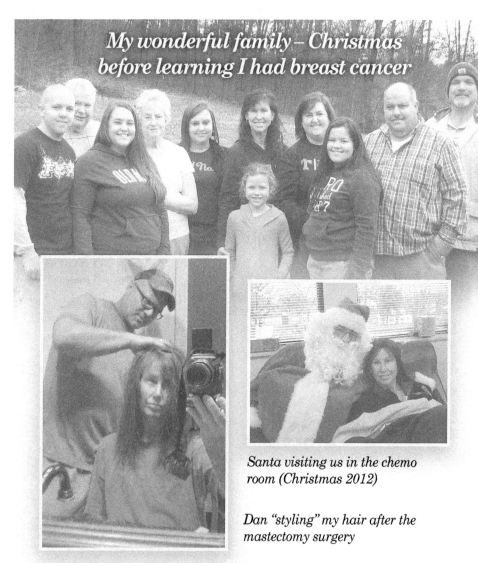

My wonderful family – Christmas before learning I had breast cancer

Santa visiting us in the chemo room (Christmas 2012)

Dan "styling" my hair after the mastectomy surgery

Alana and me the summer I was diagnosed with breast cancer

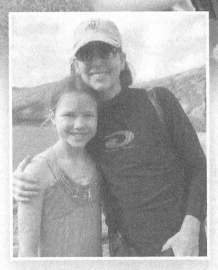

Alana and me getting ready to snorkel in Hanauma Bay (Hawaii)

Alana visiting me in the hospital after intestinal reconstruction (2013)

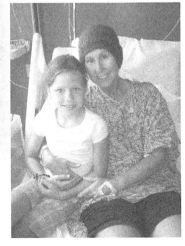

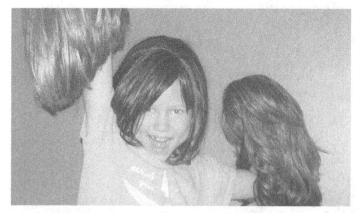

Alana having fun with my new "hair"

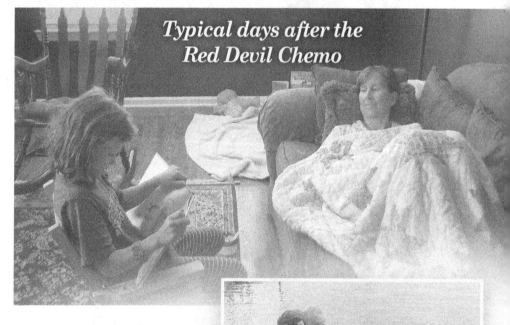

Typical days after the Red Devil Chemo

Alana and me – Halloween fun (2014)

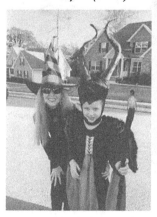

Fun times with my dad and Alana (Summer 2012)

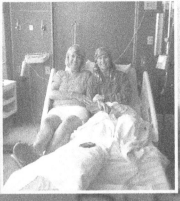

*Aunt Linda and me
after one of my surgeries*

*Good times at
Disney World –
after the roller
coaster "issue"*

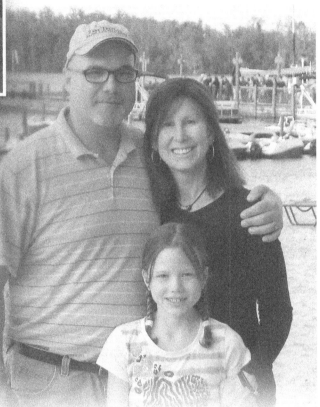

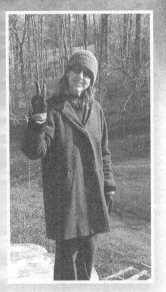

Pigeon Forge with my mom (September 2012)

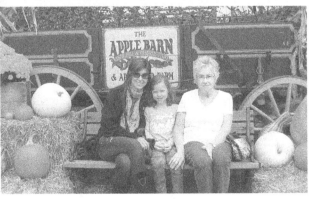

*We went back to the
state park a year after
the accident*

"A cheerful heart is good medicine, but a crushed spirit dries up the bones."
Proverbs 17:22 (NIV)

CHAPTER 17

Typical Panera Mom

Once Dan and I returned from MD Anderson, I had my third A/C treatment. The nausea started during the treatment but stayed manageable until the middle of the night. The following week continued with the same nausea, fatigue, and bone pain as the previous treatments. Thankfully, after that week and before treatment #4, mom, Alana, and I enjoyed a long weekend in Pigeon Forge. If you are in the midst of treatments, you understand that one week can be debilitating and the next almost as if you had never been sick. Then it's time for the next round, but remember, you will feel better.

Each of the four A/C treatments was delayed for various reasons (infection, illness, etc.) but I finally finished my last round of the Adriamycin/Cytoxan combination. They don't call Adriamycin (Doxorubicin is the generic name) the Red Devil for nothing. The severe side effects were cumulative and by the last of the four treatments, the nausea and pain continued well into the second week. Following those treatments, I began what would be twelve treatments of Paclitaxel.

Compared to the A/C, Paclitaxel side effects were minimal. After each treatment I would rest, but the next day I felt strong enough to manage all of our usual daily activities. Life was good. During the twelve weeks of treatment with Paclitaxel, I often referred to myself as the typical Panera mom. I could be eating lunch in Panera (one of my favorites) and no one would suspect I had been in the chemo chair the day before or that I was waiting to hear the results of my recent brain scan (that's another story). We look like any other woman attempting to eat healthy while enjoying time with friends. The next time you're in a group of people look around and remember, we never know what the person sitting close to us is going through in their life. Maybe that's why we are given seemingly simple instructions to "be kind to one another" (Ephesians 4:32).

While it was a relief to end my relationship with the Red Devil, Paclitaxel treatments included large doses of steroids. Before starting the new drug, I asked my local oncologist and my MD Anderson physician if the steroids were used to control side effects or increase the effectiveness of the chemotherapy. My plan was to reduce the steroid dose if possible. I learned the steroids were used to reduce the likelihood of a reaction, meaning I could reduce the dosage after the first few treatments if I did not have a reaction to the chemo. I started my first treatment on November 5 with the full steroid dosage. After the first three treatments, without a reaction, I was able to gradually reduce the amount of steroids. If you are concerned about steroid side effects talk with your doctor. Never change or omit any of the prescribed medications without confirmation and supervision from your oncologist.

Though I no longer struggled with nausea or other major physical side effects, I still battled fear. As I drew closer to the end of chemotherapy, reality set in. I was elated to finish chemo but worried because I would no longer have the weekly reassurance my blood levels were normal. I learned follow-up visits, labs, and exams were only once a quarter. For the past six months, chemo treatments and blood work had been a weekly part of my life, now I would have labs and exams only four times a year. This knowledge would require some adjustment time.

During one of my office visits with my oncologist, I asked when exams would begin. She said they routinely start once treatment was complete. I felt it would be helpful to have a baseline knowledge of my "new" body before the end of chemo, so I asked for an examination. I held my breath as she felt the lymph nodes under my arms. I worried she would find something suspicious. Thankfully, she did not. We then discussed the persistent pain on my lower left side. Once diagnosed with cancer, even the slightest tinge of pain can set us on high alert. We no longer have the luxury of "just" a headache or any other slight pain. Each twinge can bring with it the fear of recurrence. Since being diagnosed with cancer, I dreaded the time when I would need a scan or any other diagnostic test. I felt almost faint when my oncologist suggested I have a hip x-ray later that day.

A week passed without a call regarding my x-ray results. I prayed and read scripture to find peace. When I returned for my seventh treatment I asked the nurse for a copy of the results. Not understanding the magnitude the piece of paper held, she casually handed over the report. Tears came to my eyes as she told me it was fine. I closed my eyes and, again, thanked God. My mom asked why I was upset but she didn't pursue an answer. I had not told my parents. I wanted to spare them the additional worry.

Life remained normal during most of the Paclitaxel treatments. The discomfort in my hip continued and the body aches increased with each treatment but, compared to the A/C effects, these were manageable. We had a wonderful Christmas and enjoyed quality time with our family and friends. I completed my eighth treatment prior to the New Year. Six months had passed since my diagnosis. Six months filled with surgeries, tests, procedures, and treatments. Half a year spent relying solely on God for healing and growing deeper in my faith. I've been asked if the time went by quickly. In some ways six months had passed quickly but, at the same time, it still seemed surreal. It felt as if time stopped at certain moments. Looking into 2013, I faced four more treatments and would then be finished with chemo. The thought was both exhilarating and frightening.

January 8, 2013, I met with my oncologist prior to treatment #9. She examined the fluid pocket that had developed below my port and determined it had less fluid than the week before. As she felt under my arm she found an "irritated" lymph node about the size of a pea. She said she didn't think it was anything but, "given my history", she ordered an ultrasound. I could hear her talking but I wasn't present emotionally. I heard her say she didn't think it was cancer. My heart felt as though it might stop. There it was, that word I hate. In just a few short hours I would see my surgeon for an ultrasound, exam, and possible biopsy.

As I entered the treatment room, it took every ounce of energy and will power to hold back the tears. As I sat waiting for the nurse to numb my port I looked around the room allowing negative thoughts to consume me. I thought of all the pain and suffering everyone in those chairs had endured. I felt as though the walls might close in on me. I wanted to run from that room and everything it represented. But I sat quietly in my chair.

Those who have never walked this path cannot fully comprehend the fear. As traumatic as the mastectomy, blood clots, second surgery, transfusions, throat abscess, nausea, and bone pain were, the emotional torture is worse. I knew I needed to go to God's word for comfort but I did not.

January 23, 2013, I finished the last of my 16 chemotherapy treatments. The range of emotions that day brought were far too many to name. During the last treatment, the nurses asked if I wanted to wear the crown signifying my last treatment. I thanked them but declined. I did not want to draw attention to myself. Rather, I chose to sit in my chair as I had the past few months, chat with those around me, and soak in my surroundings.

I would not miss sitting in that reclining chair several hours a week, but I would miss the people. I developed friendships with some of the most incredible people. I would miss our weekly conversations. Without exception, every chemo nurse that administered treatment was extremely kind, hardworking, and knowledgeable. I am thankful to have had such compassionate nurses.

In my attempt to keep life's activities going through all the treatments, I accomplished my greatest claim to fame with our hike through Cloudland Canyon. Two days before my last chemo treatment, I hiked to the bottom of Cloudland Canyon State Park with Alana and friends. Nature is one of God's greatest gifts. When times are tough or good, being outside has been, and continues to be, therapeutic. When you are struggling with side effects or fear or when life is absolutely wonderful, I highly recommend taking the time to appreciate all the beauty nature has to offer.

Shortly after my last treatment I had another unexpected event. Dan managed to plan, organize, and orchestrate a surprise party. The planning, skill, and secrecy it took to accomplish all he did made the party so very special. The gathering was a beautiful celebration of life shared with family and life-long friends. The party was reminiscent of the impromptu party thrown in my living room the night before my first surgery, only this time we were rejoicing what many call survivorship status. I was happy to celebrate and glad that phase had ended. I also knew my journey was not over. Now it was time to live with the reality of healing under the new label "survivor."

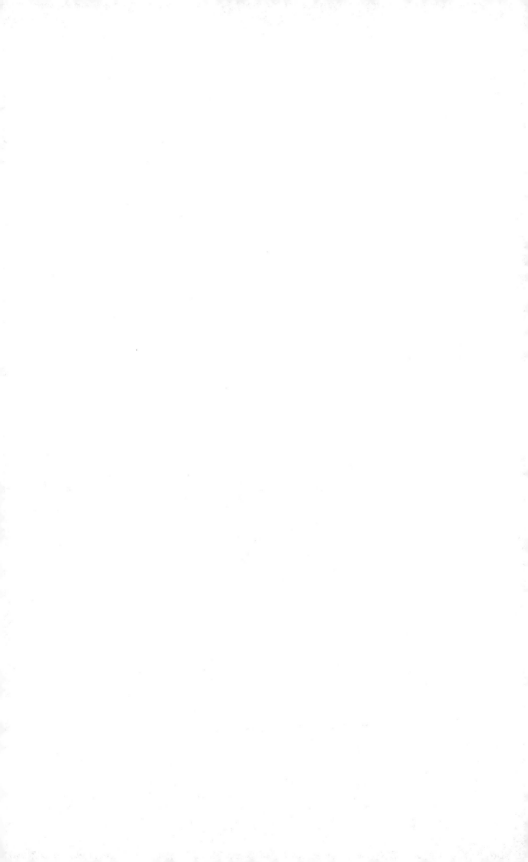

- PART IV -

Post-Treatment

"Let's suppose you had a bank that each morning credited your account $1,440 – with one condition: Whatever part of the $1,440 you had failed to use during the day would be erased from your account, and no balance would be carried over. What would you do? You'd draw out every cent every day and use it to your best advantage. Well, you do have such a bank, and its name is time. Every morning this bank credits you with 1,440 minutes. And it writes off as forever lost whatever portion you have failed to invest in good purpose."
Author Unknown

CHAPTER 18

The Wonderful World of Uneventful // Prognosis… "Good"

The first month after treatment ends can feel like a total whirlwind. We transition from seeing our doctor frequently to only a few times a year. Be prepared, adjusting to the survivorship phase of a cancer diagnosis takes time both physically and mentally. When you finish treatment, you will most likely go through a survivorship meeting with either your nurse navigator or nurse practitioner. In this meeting he or she will go over a summary of your diagnosis, treatment, and prognosis (more on this word a little later).

While follow-up appointments are an important and necessary part of post-treatment life, there are other factors that go into life after cancer. PearlPoint Cancer Support offers a free Survivorship Handbook on their website that has in-depth guidance on how to live a healthy, preventative, and stress-free (does that really exist?) life once treatment is complete. The following are just a few points taken from the handbook, but you can visit their website to find all these points and more in detail[10].

Nutrition and Healthy Lifestyle – Cancer treatments take a big toll on your body. Healthy post-treatment nutritional and lifestyle choices not only give your body a chance to restore what was lost, but they can also play a huge part in preventing recurrence.

- Include a variety of colorful fruits and vegetables into your daily diet. If something is not seasonal, frozen fruits and vegetables are a good alternative to fresh.
- Eating complex carbohydrates such as whole grains can increase your energy levels.
- Choose lean protein – eggs, white meat, beans – over red meat.
- Drink lots of water.

- Continue to clean raw foods well and cook food thoroughly before eating.
- Maintain an active lifestyle. Exercising for at least 45 minutes a day helps you maintain a healthy weight, which plays a role in cancer prevention. Remember not to overdo your exercise or work too hard too fast. Exercise should be done in moderation—remember the goal is to be healthy.

Managing Long-Term Side Effects – While some of your side effects from treatment may disappear once treatment ends, there are some potential side effects that may remain depending on your type of treatment. Below are just a few side effects you could experience past treatment and how to deal with them. If you experience these or any other unusual symptoms, you should always tell your doctor. Remember, your doctor can't help you if they don't know.

- *Heart damage* – Some radiation and chemo treatments have been shown to cause minor heart damage and increase the possibility of cardiac issues. One of the best ways to manage and counteract this side effect is through a healthy diet and exercise.
- *Chemo brain* – After going through chemotherapy, you may experience trouble remembering certain things or have trouble concentrating. Many refer to this as "chemo brain." This can be long-term or short-term depending on the individual and cause of the side effect (i.e. treatment drug, etc.). There are many ways to manage chemo brain, such as keeping lists and writing down reminders, staying well-rested physically and mentally, eating well, staying active, and exercising your mind with puzzles or logic games.
- *Fatigue* – You may feel an overall sense of tiredness after finishing treatment. The normal response to fatigue is to rest, but too much rest can actually make you more tired. In order to counteract fatigue, stay active and eat energy-boosting foods that fuel your body.

Getting back to normal – After a life-threatening diagnosis your health gets thrown into the spotlight and you go into autopilot mode. After treatment, however, your mind gets a chance to slow down and it's important not to remain on autopilot but return to life as normally as you can. If you stopped working after the diagnosis, returning to normal may look like going back to work. Whatever your normal, make sure you take time to process and pursue this next phase gradually.

Checking for signs of recurrence – Recurrence is not a fun word, but going to your follow-up appointments and knowing the symptoms of recurrence are an important aspect of post-treatment life. Ask your doctor what you should keep an eye on, such as unusual body pain or bleeding/discharge from the breast or any other persistent symptom. An easy way to keep alert to symptoms is by doing a self-check each month for lumps in the breast. If you experience anything unusual physically or emotionally, always tell your doctor.

The weeks following the last chemo treatment went by rather uneventfully, which is an adjective I truly didn't appreciate enough until it was gone. Life went about almost as it had before the diagnosis—no more trips to the chemo room and the nausea was gone. My body was slowly recovering from chemo and adjusting to this new normal.

February 2013, three weeks after chemo, we took a much-needed family vacation to Disney World. It was a truly wonderful vacation. We traveled with friends and had a fun-filled time together. Watching Alana meet the characters, ride thrilling rides, and simply enjoy being a kid was, as they say in Disney, absolutely magical. I was so happy to be able to enjoy this trip so soon after treatment ended.

Following our trip to Disney, I started follow-up appointments with both my surgeon and oncologist. During an appointment with my oncologist, we discussed the standard timeline for keeping the chemo port. Typically, patients wait two years before having the port removed. I wasn't sure I wanted to wait that long. She explained 80% of recurrences happen within the first two years. There it was again... another dreaded statistic. I sat there wishing I had not heard that comment. We discussed the possibility of removing it sooner. I am an optimist and chose to believe I would no longer need the port but agreed to wait and make the decision later. Once I was alone in the room, I did as I would many more times in the months to come; I knelt beside the exam table and thanked God for healing.

The next day I met with my oncologist's nurse practitioner for what they refer to as the "survivorship meeting." She went over a summary of my diagnosis, treatment, and follow-up. The first page of the document described my original diagnosis followed by my prognosis. My breath stopped as I read the sentence: "prognosis... (drum roll in my head)... good." A surge of relief rushed over me and I actually laughed out loud. I explained the laughter was relief knowing I now had it in writing that my future looked "good." She smiled but I'm not certain she understood the magnitude of the conversation.Another physician once said "our future is 100% or 0%". I agree. Our prognosis is always "good." We are alive right now. God has a purpose for this minute of our lives. It is our responsibility to fill those minutes in a way that honors Him.

GLIMPSES, VISIONS, AND HOPE

"And my God will meet all your needs according to the riches of his glory in Christ Jesus."

Philippians 4:19

Sometimes God supplies hope when we need Him the most. His promises can be sent through many different channels including glimpses of our future. I have enjoyed reading of others' visions of the future or glimpses of heaven but, He had not allowed me to personally experience either until I was deeply grieving the loss of my friend. Shortly after my cancer diagnosis, I met a precious lady who was also being treated for triple negative breast cancer. Lisa was a constant encourager and spirit of light in my life. She fought with everything she had and ultimately God chose to heal her and take her to live with Him. The day I learned Lisa had passed away I was consumed with grief. I lay across the bed sobbing with Dan on one side and Alana on the other. I cried for a long time but at one point, through my tears, I remember vividly seeing a vision of myself very old. I was in a wheelchair and Alana was standing behind me. I wasn't thrilled about the wheelchair but I was filled with hope that I would have a future. I know some will argue our brain produces visuals to calm us (I would have argued this in the past) but Isaiah 40:29 tells us, "He gives strength to the weary." Jesus wants to give us what we need the very moment we need if we only ask.

Jesus allowed another vision of hope a little later. Alana and I had recently attended a bridal shower and while enjoying the festivities the thought, "I might not be here when Alana gets married", hit me like the proverbial brick wall. I was suddenly so upset I had to go to the bathroom to talk and pray my way through the anxiety. Later, Jesus gave me a brief picture of Alana at, what appeared to be, her bridal shower. She sat in the middle of a room wearing a blue dress and looked absolutely beautiful. I thank God for this glimpse of hope as I struggled through the "what if" fears. As you continue through this cancer journey terrifying thoughts can grip you when you least expect them. Call on Jesus; ask Him to give you exactly what you need in that moment.

The last event (that I am consciously aware of) came in the spring of 2013. I was sitting alone on our deck enjoying the warm afternoon sun when I saw an older version of Dan walking up toward me from a lake. There was a framed swing beside the water but that's all I could remember. We had always wanted lake property but at that time had not found anything affordable (especially with our budget). In the fall of 2015 we stumbled across a piece of property on the lake that we could actually afford. This purchase made that glance feel more real, but then I questioned, "Why did I need to actually own the property before I believed the vision came from God?" This question led to another thought: "Now that we own this property, am I closer to death?" "Is this vision coming true now and I really won't live to be old?" Satan will do everything possible to cause us to doubt that God truly wants to give us "hope and a future" (Jeremiah 29:11). John 10:10 (ESV) tells us "The thief comes only to steal and kill and destroy." Jesus came not only to give us life but to give us an abundant life. He doesn't want us to just survive; He wants us to enjoy an abundant life. When challenges seem insurmountable ask Him for the strength, hope, and courage you need.

These flashes of the future gave me hope that I would grow old with my husband and live many more years with Alana. I wish I could write that God continually blessed me with visions but I cannot. However, I wonder… does He give us these peeks into our future but we're too busy to notice or we chalk them up to coincidence or just a passing thought? Maybe that's why He tells us "to be still and know that I am God" (Psalms 46:10).

*****

The one-year anniversary of my diagnosis came June 11, 2013. One year prior my doctor called to tell me the biopsy results were positive for breast cancer. On that day the rough journey began. Though it had been a year of anxiety and indescribable fear, I could also see the blessings that sprang from the diagnosis. On June 15 we went with friends to Dollywood's Splash Country Water Park. The last time we were there was the weekend before I received that life-changing phone call. Little did I know then that I would return a year later completely transformed and even more grateful for every precious moment of life.

Along with the anniversary of my diagnosis, the summer also marked the one-year anniversary of my healing, June 21, 2013. God had allowed my primary care doctor and surgeon to be a part of this miraculous healing. As I looked back over the past year, I couldn't believe all that had happened. There were times post-treatment when I could still feel the blow of hearing "you have cancer." The thought, "I had cancer," could occur anywhere, when I least expected it. There were times when I hoped I might still wake from a dream. A dream filled with many negative emotions but also positives, most of all my new closer relationship with Jesus and an even greater appreciation for life than I had previously known.

While some of my notes from diagnosis through post-treatment deal with fear or suffering, the vast majority of my life was (and is) filled with joy and contentment. Prior to the diagnosis I loved life and that continues with a heightened awareness and appreciation for simply being alive. After encountering a life-threatening event, I've heard people talk about an acute awareness of the beauty around them, the smell of flowers, and so on. This is true but, thankfully, I was grateful for God's extreme gifts prior to the diagnosis. Someone would have to look long and hard to find anyone who loves life more.

In April we visited a friend's church to celebrate her daughter's baptism. The minister made an excellent point that truly resonated with me. He said healing miracles are not about the healing but about showing the power of God. As I thought about his statement, I tried connecting the dots of the past couple years. "Was this why I had triple negative?" "Does God want me to speak about His healing power?" "Was I being used as a vessel to demonstrate His modern day healing?" Previously when I had read or listened to others talk I had sometimes wondered why did I have to get the "bad" type? "Why did I need to have chemo?" I knew I needed to hold these thoughts captive but they remained as I wrestled with understanding the purpose behind the pain. Even if only in the recesses of our mind, we all want to know the purpose behind our suffering. Admittedly, I am such a weak vessel. I am afraid if I had been diagnosed with something "mild" (though no such cancer exists) I might not have relied on God to the extent I now do.

Even though my treatments were over, my reliance on God was challenged every single day. When I attempted to face this journey alone; when I questioned why; when I didn't read God's word; when I didn't consistently pray—the fear returned. It was when I gave God all the credit, spoke of His healing power, and practiced the faith He speaks of throughout His Word that I was blessed with the most gloriously peaceful and content feelings, all of which is still true today.

*****

Mark 11:24, Matthew 7:7-11, James 4:3, John 14:13-14, John 15:7, instruct us to "ask." We are to ask Jesus for healing, for peace, for all needs. We are told to take all our requests to Him. Mark 11:24-25 tells us to ask, believe, and forgive. When I first learned I had cancer I mastered the art of asking, I begged. Later I learned Jesus instructed us to bring our requests to Him, to believe He will answer our prayer, and then He goes on to tell us we must forgive anything we hold against another person.

After the initial shock of learning I had cancer, I clung to these promises. I truly believe Jesus wants us to ask and then believe He will provide. When Jesus came to his hometown he performed less miracles there than anywhere because they did not believe. We must have faith. This takes us back to the question we will either silently or verbally want to know—why do some people survive and others do not? I certainly do not claim to have the answer. But I can say, as someone who has struggled with the very real fear of dying, I do believe, regardless of the outcome, He never leaves us nor forsakes us.

"The Lord is my light and my salvation — whom shall I fear? The Lord is the stronghold of my life — of whom shall I be afraid?"
Psalm 27:1 (NIV)

CHAPTER 19

Genetic Testing[6]

For some, genetic testing is the epitome of the phrase "knowledge is power." For others, testing would bring only more worry and fear. Neither is right or wrong, we each must decide what is best in our circumstances. Though not much is involved physically with testing – it only requires a blood or saliva sample – it can add another difficult emotional decision to be made in the midst of a recent cancer diagnosis.

While meeting with the physician for a second opinion at MD Anderson, she told me that there could be a genetic component involved and that I might want to consider genetic testing. Though the probability was low, I wanted to know the likelihood that I could have passed a gene mutation to Alana and/or her future children.

Gene mutations are changes in the genetic code, the part of your DNA that literally makes you the way you are. While most mutations happen during a person's lifetime with no known cause, some mutations can be passed down from generation to generation. In the United States only about 5-10% of breast cancers are caused by an inherited gene mutation. The best known breast cancer gene mutations are BRCA 1 and BRCA 2, which are also linked to ovarian cancer. It is important to note that these mutations do not guarantee breast cancer development but simply increase one's risk of being diagnosed. Some with BRCA 1/2 never get breast cancer and, in fact, most diagnoses are not linked to the mutation at all.

Before being tested for any breast cancer gene mutation, you must go through genetic counseling with a professional. The counselor will first speak with you about your family history to determine if there is a need for the test. Those most at risk for carrying the mutation are women with an immediate connection to breast cancer, such as the diagnosis of a mother, father (though less likely, men can also have breast cancer), sister, or daughter. Usually the diagnosed family member is tested first. If no gene mutation is found in someone with breast cancer, it could be inferred they didn't pass down the mutation to family members.

If your family history does show a need for testing, the genetic counselor will explain all that goes along with testing. Topics of discussion will include the medical cost of testing, the emotional risk and impact of the test, and what you plan to do with the results. Once these are covered, a blood or saliva sample is taken and sent away for analysis. Your genetic counselor will then review and explain the results of the test. These test results can come back one of three ways:

- *Negative/Normal* – no mutation found
- *Positive/Carrier* – mutation linked to breast cancer found
- *Variant/Uncertain Significance* – mutation not currently known to increase breast cancer risk found[11]

Another genetic test that goes further than the BRACAnalysis (BRCA 1/2 test) is the BRACAnalysis Large Rearrangement Test (BART). BART was created by Myriad to detect genetic rearrangements not found with the previous test. Even though these arrangements account for 6-10% of hereditary mutations for breast and ovarian cancer, the BART is more difficult to get approved than typical genetic testing. In order for BART to be included as part of the BRACAnalysis with no additional charge, the National Comprehensive Cancer Network (NCCN) has come up with criteria that must be met. The criteria, in short, states that anyone wanting BART to be covered by insurance or as part of the typical genetic test must have a specific, very strong family history of the disease. If you are BRCA 1/2 positive this certainly does not guarantee a future cancer diagnosis, only that you are statistically at an increased risk. Most importantly, discuss all statistics, family history, and options with your medical treatment team[12].

Genetic testing can give you a plethora of knowledge while also bringing an abundance of choices. Fear and uncertainties can also be attached to this new found knowledge. Because it is not set in stone you will develop breast cancer if you have the gene mutation, you have to weigh the physical and emotional benefits and risks of testing. As you should with all medical decisions, speak with your treatment team regarding the pros and cons of genetic testing.

"Have I gone mad?" asked the Mad Hatter.
"I'm afraid so," replied Alice. "You're entirely bonkers.
But I'll tell you a secret. All the best people are."
Alice in Wonderland (2010 movie)

CHAPTER 20

Body and Mind Connection

"What just happened?" "Am I going crazy?" "My body is out of control!" "How can I have cancer when I feel fine?" These are all normal thoughts that you may experience throughout your cancer journey. I certainly had all of these and many more. These thoughts can make us feel crazy or, as Alice said, entirely bonkers.

While it's normal to have these feelings we must battle to keep the thoughts passing through and not lingering. Keeping your body nourished during treatment is important but you need to also focus on keeping another part of your body healthy—your mind. Mental health has a major impact on your physical condition. Whether your thoughts are positive or negative they can influence your health, so it's important to do things during your treatment that cater to rejuvenating your mind and spirit. The following tips are from a licensed therapist who specializes in working with oncology clients:

- Connect with a support group or cancer resource center. Try different scenarios until you find one that fits your personality – one-on-one, small groups, larger groups, etc.
- Reach out to others. Plenty of resources can usually be found in the hospital where you're being treated. If not, reach out to other local hospitals and cancer resource centers.
- Connect with others who share your diagnosis.
- Be open-minded to alternative therapy options – acupuncture, mindfulness, and other options – in conjunction with your treatment plan.
- A cancer diagnosis is traumatic to the body and mind, it can also cause past emotional or physical traumas to resurface. This is one of the times when you might feel those, "Am I crazy" emotions, but be assured, those

are normal thoughts. Find a therapist to help you sort through the memories and their accompanying emotions.

- You may feel ambushed by your grief, and sometimes it will be accompanied by guilt from comparing yourself to others. This is YOUR grief. Don't compare it to anyone else's, no matter your situation.

- There will be a shift in who you are, but this can be a positive experience. Even though you may not be able to see it in the present moment, the valleys of life can lead to positive peaks.

- Nurture yourself. Ask yourself what nurturing looks like to you and then do it. Don't let others dictate how you should take care of yourself.
  - *For example,* being outside soothes me. I need to be outdoors as often as possible. During treatment my dad bought me a nice chair and fluffy cushion for my deck so I could enjoy the privacy and being outside. When I felt especially daring, I would sit on the deck and enjoy the warm sunshine on my bald head. At least I did until I remembered Google Earth could be videoing. Darn Google Earth!

- From the time of your diagnosis and throughout treatment, there will be times when you feel as though you are living on auto pilot—you are. Accept it and trust yourself to make the best possible decisions during those times.

- Try to understand there will be moments when you live in a spirit of fear, but don't stay there. Accept your situation, understand its implications, and then go forward with a positive, healthy mindset.

- Remember we all have those passing thoughts of "what will happen when I'm gone" but don't allow them to linger. These thoughts only feed our fear.

- You don't have to be a "good patient." Most of us want to be a compliant patient but that doesn't mean we shouldn't ask questions. If you have a concern or don't understand any part of your treatment plan, ask questions. Your team members can't help if they don't know there is a problem.

- Don't second guess what you think is best for you. Everything is happening so fast. Take in all the information you've been given and then make a decision. Move forward knowing you made the best possible decision.

- Avoid comparing yourself to others (we should practice this one all the time regardless of our circumstances).

One evening Alana and I both were struggling with comparisons so we talked extensively about the pitfalls of comparing. We agreed that if I compared my bald head to someone else's long, beautiful hair I would feel terrible. We determined that pitting our life and circumstances against anyone is an unfair comparison and only makes us feel bad. Ann Voskamp said it best: "Measuring sticks always become weapons... Pick up a yardstick to measure your life against anyone else's and you've just picked up a stick and beaten up your soul."

A cancer diagnosis is a traumatic experience both physically and mentally. Some women who don't need radiation, reconstruction, or chemotherapy may go through stages of guilt questioning why they feel so bad when others have it much worse. This is normal. Other women look at those with metastatic breast cancer and feel guilty for fearing recurrence. In short, everyone is always worried because someone out there has it worse than them. Remember, your pain is your pain and can only be compared to the experiences of your own life. Stephen Chbosky wrote, "And even if somebody else has it much worse, that doesn't really change the fact that you have what you have" (Perks of Being a Wallflower, 2012). It's easy to slip into the void of "they have it worse/better than me", but avoid this mindset and commend others for fighting their fight while also recognizing your own.

*****

The roller coaster of emotions that follow any life-altering diagnosis can be exhausting and exhilarating. Hang on; this roller coaster may bring a depth of fear never before known, but it can also give you an opportunity to experience relief and joy greater than any other time in your life. Below are a few excerpts from my original journal showing the range of emotions experienced daily and sometimes hourly. If you see yourself in any of these, know you're not crazy... or maybe we both are, but either way the coaster continues.

> *Five days ago* I learned I have breast cancer. As Alana quietly slept, I knelt beside her bed again tonight and begged God to let me live. I imagined her life without me. I thought of dying. I thought of the grief Alana would go through. I can't believe this is happening. I curled up on the floor sobbing, begging God for my life. Over and over I pleaded, "Please don't take me from her."

> *Four months ago* I learned I have breast cancer. This weekend Mom, Alana, and I went on one of our wonderful trips to Pigeon Forge in between chemo treatments. Awesome weekend!

> *April 1, 2013:* I watched my precious baby sleep tonight. I begged God to allow me to watch her grow up.

> *April 19, 2013:* My surgeon said everything appeared completely normal. After he left the room, I got on my knees beside the exam table and thanked God.

> *August 2013:* I just scheduled the dreaded bone scan. Today is Tuesday, the scan is Friday. I am numb with fear. I want to curl up in a corner and cry but tears won't come. I dread waiting for the scan results, what if I'm dying, what if the cancer has spread, what if I don't have long to live. Now the tears are coming.

November 2013: Life is somewhat normal. I have always appreciated "normal." I now love "normal."

April 2014: Torture, torture, torture! That's the only word to describe the feelings when I allow my thoughts to enter that horrible place.

May 2014: I'm concerned the only time I write is when I'm upset or dealing with fear. The vast majority of my life is filled with joy, laughter, and good times.

July 2014: My friend went to live with Jesus. She fought with everything she had to live. She was one of the most dedicated Christians I have ever known. She was an amazing mom, wife, daughter, and friend. I miss her so much.

December 2016: I'll be so glad when this book is finished.

January 2017: As Alana and I were driving down our hill, a huge tree limb fell and smashed into our car. Glass went everywhere. Thankfully, Alana was in the backseat and we're both ok. But how many freaky things can happen to a person in a lifetime? Thank you, God, again, for always staying with us.

"I have loved the stars too fondly to be fearful of the night."
Galileo

CHAPTER 21

Controlling the "What If" Monster // Scripture and Cupcakes are a Powerful Combination

As I mentioned in the introduction, I write of the fears, struggles and challenges hoping to help those going through any life altering event know these thoughts are normal. More importantly, to help them know the peace that comes when we turn all the anxiety, fear, and any other negative emotion to Jesus. As I look back over the first two years since the cancer diagnosis, I realize I experienced a level of fear I had never known. I also experienced joy in the greatest and purest form. We all struggle with fear but for many different reasons. In hindsight I realized that during the first two years after learning I had cancer, I lived somewhat in a fog. I certainly did not know this during that time but, now that the fog is beginning to lift, I know I struggled far too often with fear. Satan gives us just enough truth mixed into his lies to induce doubt and fear. He can tell us "your friend died, you will too." "You can't overcome this, no one can." "The doctors said other people only live X number of months or years, you'll be the same." He may give a fragment of truth to snag our attention, but we must always remember that he is the father of lies and the master of deceit.

Psalm 23:4 gives us a depiction of fear I often associate with my story: "Yea, though I walk through the valley of the shadow of death, I will fear no evil; For You are with me; Your rod and Your staff, they comfort me" (NKJV). On one side you have a large, looming grim reaper hovering over a tiny, frail individual (. . . though I walk through the valley of the shadow of death . . .). I often saw myself as that frail person. But on the other side you have sunrays shining down on this same person with hope from God (. . . . will fear no evil, for you are with me . . .). In times of fear remember, God says we walk through the valley, meaning the valley has an end. We are coming out on the other side.

Controlling the fear a cancer diagnosis brings is one of our greatest struggles. The initial shock of learning we have cancer puts us into fight mode. The year following treatment can also bring its own set of challenges. After I finished chemo,

I was asked repeatedly when the scans would begin. Most people, myself included, assumed I would have CT scans or some other test to be certain the cancer had not returned. This is not the case. The NCCN guidelines state exams are to be done during follow-up visits with your doctor between one and four times a year (about every three months) for the first five years. Upon your sixth year post-treatment, your visits decrease to once a year unless you develop new symptoms. Even further, these guidelines also state imaging tests are not required in those who underwent bilateral mastectomy and/or had reconstructive surgery for stages 1 and 2[13]. However, those diagnosed with stage 3 are recommended to receive a mammogram every year[14]. These guidelines are subject to change over time, which is why you should talk with your treatment team about scans, mammograms, and any other diagnostic testing and always tell your doctor of any new, unusual, or persistent symptoms.

During chemotherapy the normal routine is to see a doctor or nurse before each treatment. I went from talking with my oncologist or the nurse practitioner weekly to getting checked once every three months. I (somewhat) jokingly told my oncologist that I felt like the dumped girlfriend. I had been kicked to the medical curb. I was glad weekly appointments were no longer necessary, but it was emotionally difficult to transition from knowing exactly what my blood counts were each week to waiting three months before the next appointment. Although physical exams and seeing your oncologist and/or surgeon becomes part of your life after a diagnosis, I took this to a whole new level. I arranged my appointments so that I had an appointment with either my surgeon or my oncologist every six weeks. Waiting three months in this early stage of post treatment was too long for me. This was not necessary and, in hindsight, somewhat embarrassing. I often wondered, "Why do I continually need a doctor to confirm what God has already told me." If you have recently completed treatment and have mixed emotions of relief and anxiousness, know this feeling will diminish. You will adjust to the schedule you and your doctor establish and, with time, this too will become your comfortable normal.

I am often asked if the physical pain or the emotional fear was worse. As traumatic as the bilateral mastectomy, the hematomas, second surgery, blood transfusions, throat abscess, procedure without anesthesia, nausea, staying in bed sick, and hurting for days had been, among all these the emotional torture was the worst. Unlike the body pain and nausea that went away over time, the fear and dread of "what if" lingered, at times barely present and at others the old "what if" monster loomed large.

While in treatment we are ready to fight for survival. We can't wait for all the chemo and/or radiation to be finished. But once it is all over we begin to have the time and energy to process all the emotions from the cancer diagnosis and the treatments. If you begin to feel sad or depressed at any point during or after treatment talk with your oncologist. Many cancer survivors experience depression following chemotherapy. According to the American Cancer Society, 25% of those diagnosed with cancer suffer from depression[15]. Heightened feelings of anxiety can also be seen in both male and female caregivers. Reasons for these depressive states and moments of anxiousness vary depending on individual situations, but can be caused from the strain this life-altering diagnosis puts on families. From the change of lifestyle and plans, body changes, financial issues, and the fear of death, cancer puts a heavy weight on the psyche for both those diagnosed and those who love and care for them[16].

Although I struggled after treatment, I did not experience the depression some go through. I believe it helped tremendously that, while I was taking the final rounds of chemo, we planned our first family visit to Disney World. Three weeks after finishing treatment we went to Disney with some of our closest friends. If possible, plan a trip or party or something special to enjoy once your treatment is complete. My next great adventure was also planned, one month after we returned from Disney I was scheduled to have a hysterectomy. I did not look forward to that adventure... but that's another story.

*****

When I talk with women after a life threatening diagnosis most will agree we no longer have the luxury of "just." We don't have just a headache, just a pain, or just a cough, at least not until we are several years past our diagnosis. All it takes is one pain, one discomfort, anything slightly different from the norm and we can be filled with dread. Is the cancer back? Has it spread to other parts of my body? Has something new formed? What is this pain trying to tell me?

November 2013 A few nights ago Alana came downstairs after going to bed. I knew immediately she really just needed some extra mommy time. We snuggled again and read another bible story. Shortly after leaving her room I heard her sobbing. My heart broke as I stood outside her door. In that short moment listening to her sobs I think I could have gone insane thinking of dying. of being forced to leave her.

After years of studying psychology, I knew the impact my thoughts had on how I felt physically and emotionally. Cognitive behavior therapy tells us that the way we perceive certain circumstances directly influences our feelings and actions[17]. God's word tells us "hold every thought captive" (2 Corinthians 10:5). Yet I struggled with thought control.

Irrational runaway thoughts can hit you suddenly in the most unlikely of places. This happened while we were in the "happiest place on earth" just a couple weeks after finishing chemo. Standing in one of the Disney gift shops, I noticed my right elbow was sore to the touch. Quicker than I could stop them, the thoughts flooded my mind: "Is the cancer back?" "Is it in my bones?" "What does this pain mean?" The discomfort lasted only a day, but it happened so unexpectedly that my mind instantly went to the worst possible scenario. After going through this journey, we must battle the 'what if' monster. We must not allow negative thoughts and fears to dampen any of our great, upcoming post-treatment adventures.

*****

When we think we have everything under control we can be attacked not only through our conscious thoughts but our subconscious as well. February 15, 2014, I awoke at four in the morning from a nightmare. I was a year post-treatment and life was good. I still had to work to control my thoughts but certainly was not living everyday life consumed with fear. Yet somewhere in the back of my mind remained the fear of recurrence that manifested itself that night.

In the dream I had gone for blood work and the nurse called to tell me the cancer was back. The details were fuzzy, but the results clearly showed it had metastasized throughout my body. I cried. I screamed. I instantly thought of being forced to leave Alana. She was only nine years old and I was dying. When my chest clinched so tight I could barely breathe, I was finally released from the nightmare. I laid in bed attempting to process the dream while also convincing myself it was only that—a dream. But I simply couldn't shake it. Dan tried to comfort me; he told me several of his comical dreams. Then he unexpectedly said, "Let's eat a cupcake!" I don't know what happened but I started to laugh. I laughed uncontrollably for several minutes. Once I gained my composure, I walked to the kitchen and retrieved the cupcakes. This was certainly not something I would normally do at 4:00 AM but we talked, laughed, and ate a cupcake. Before attempting sleep again, I read Matthew 9:21-22, Matthew 8:13, Matthew 5:16, Philippians 4:6-7, Proverbs 12:25, Proverbs 17:22, James 5:14-15, and Matthew 21:22. The moral of the story: cupcakes and scripture make a powerful combination.

The following is a section from my journal at the time: March 27, 2014 – I can't stop thinking of the friends I have lost to cancer and the ones who are going through treatment. I see the faces of friends no longer here; I see the faces of friends sitting in the chemo chairs week after week. We all struggle with fear while hanging on to every ounce of hope given. It's not fair! I want to scream but I know I won't. I feel guilty and truly don't want to question God because I know He is in control and loves us so very much. I know it's not my place in life to understand. I know He has a plan for everyone. But now and many times in the past and unfortunately probably more in the future I want to scream how unfair it all seems! "When will this fear go away?" "Will it ever go away?" I know I'm supposed to give all this to Jesus but I'm harboring it and I don't know what to do. My head hurts, I feel nauseated. I want to scream, "Will this fear ever end?" "Jesus forgive me for not leaning on you. Jesus I believe, please help my disbelief."

As I was writing the above I received a text from a dear friend who was so sick she could not leave her home to purchase a wig. My heart broke for her. I went to the sofa where I laid when I was sick, knelt down, and asked God to give her the warm blanket of peace that only He can give. I asked the Holy Spirit to let her feel His presence. Alana came and knelt beside me, together we prayed for each friend as they continued their fight with cancer.

Following any major diagnosis it is normal to consider all the many "what ifs" and the plethora of possibilities that could happen. I struggled most with the fear of recurrence. I sometimes forgot that God is a God of healing regardless of what our well-educated medical community predicts. Thankfully, He isn't limited to healing only certain stages of cancer or any other disease. Since first learning I had cancer, I have met many women who were diagnosed in late stages with large tumors and varying prognosis. The majority of these women are not just surviving (as they say in the post breast cancer community), they are thriving. God is with us, He is healing, He is listening, He wants to relieve our fears, He wants us to lean on Him and live a life filled with contentment and joy.

April 24, 2014 — There was a time when I did not know if I would be here to celebrate Alana's 9th or 10th birthday. Thank you, Jesus, she will be 10 tomorrow and I am here!

If you are struggling with fear, anxieties, or any of the negative emotions the enemy wants you to believe, turn to scripture. Allow God to give you the peace He so greatly desires for you to claim. Cling to His promises. Pray for His peace. Remember, He will never leave, He will never forsake you.

"She said to herself, 'If I only touch his cloak, I will be healed.' Jesus turned and saw her. 'Take heart, daughter,' he said, 'your faith has healed you.' And the woman was healed at that moment."
Matthew 9:21-22 (NIV)

CHAPTER 22

The Bone Scans

As I write of my struggles with fear I must also emphasize the vast majority of my life is not consumed with fear. I am blessed with a husband that loves me, an amazing daughter, wonderful parents, family, and friends. I chose to disclose the scares and the fear-filled events after the diagnosis in an attempt to help those going through this journey understand each of the emotions felt are normal. The joy is real, probably the greatest I've ever felt. The fear is also real. I am transparent about my fear-driven decisions in order to help others discern between a real need and an irrational fear-based decision. I made some of both.

Since the initial diagnosis, I have dreaded the time when a scan would be necessary. I often told Dan I didn't know if I could handle the anxiety of any type of scan. I do not fear the machine, the process, or anything related to the procedure, but I fear the results the scan could disclose. Most women I've interviewed agree it's the fear of the unknown that is maddening.

August 2013, fourteen months after my diagnosis, I told my oncologist my back had been uncomfortable. I made excuses—working out, sleeping in an odd position, etc. I explained it wasn't painful but the discomfort had continued for a few months. She immediately said she would order a bone scan. There it was, that horrible, dreaded word "scan." I asked if we could just order an x-ray of my lower back rather than a bone scan. She explained the x-ray would not be as thorough and for my peace of mind, and to rule out any "bad cells," I should have the scan. I dreaded that scan as if I were going to slowly have my skin removed . . . that might be a slight exaggeration but only slight.

August 23, 2013, Dan and I arrived at the hospital for my first bone scan. As part of the imaging prep, I had an injection three hours prior to the start of the scan. Thankfully, the injection is painless. While waiting for the scan, we went to lunch at a quaint restaurant with outdoor seating, simply being outside helped to lower my anxiety. I thought of how "normal" we must appear; just another couple enjoying lunch. Although this was not just another lunch, it helped relieve some of the stress of waiting for the scan. I managed to eat. Unfortunately, almost nothing stops my appetite. I recommend going somewhere you enjoy during the time between the injection and the scan. Those three hours can feel endless, make this time as pleasurable as possible. Dan was trying to make me laugh but I know he was worried too. I worry so much I convinced him to worry too—great gift I have.

When we returned to the hospital, I had fought back the tears almost as long as I could. I took shallow breathes and felt there could be a breakdown coming. I'm not sure what this breakdown would look like but I felt it looming.

Once in the room, the technician began explaining the procedure. He said the scan would take approximately 30 minutes unless additional testing was required but he didn't think that would be necessary. I wondered what he based that statement on since the scan hadn't even started yet, however I wanted to believe him. I was convinced if additional tests were needed something was terribly wrong.

He went on to say the machine would come very close but would not touch my face or body. As he finished the instructions, I told both technicians I was wearing a wig but had a hat to wear during the scan. They were so kind, they graciously told me they wouldn't have known it was a wig and left the room so I could change. My hands shook as I fumbled through changing into the gown and my hat. Then it was time for the scan to begin.

I felt my body trembling, almost vibrating, as the machine started, yet somehow I managed to remain perfectly still. I worried that if I moved it would interfere with the scan results. My irrational thoughts told me if the results came back clear after scanning my trembling body, they could be inaccurate. My adrenaline was so extreme I could not focus. I feared I might pass out. I feared I might start screaming and not be able to stop. I feared if I started to cry the tears would become uncontrollable. I feared I might do all of these and wake up committed to my local mental health facility. Thankfully, none of this happened. I somehow managed to control my shaking limbs and irrational thoughts.

I tried to recall scripture as the scan continued. I certainly don't claim to be well-versed with memorized scripture but I do have several favorites that I can usually recall. However, I could only remember one verse: "Be of good cheer, daughter; your faith has made you well" (Matthew 9:22 NKJV). This single verse ran repeatedly through my thoughts as the machine slowly scanned my body. I blamed my high adrenaline for the memory lapse, but later realized Jesus gave me that single verse in the very moment I needed it most.

BONE SCAN #2

Dan and I ate at a local restaurant during the waiting period after the injection. Looking around at the other people enjoying their lunch, I realized no one would ever guess that I was waiting to return to the hospital for a scan that could produce life-changing results. Watching everyone reinforced my belief that we can never truly know what the person next to us is going through. Again, I looked like anyone else eating lunch. No one could possibly have known the fear I was struggling to suppress.

It wasn't long before the nurse called me back. The technician was a beautiful lady who was pregnant with her first child. We talked about babies and the joy of becoming a mom. I told her when I became a mom I felt a love that, prior to having my daughter, I didn't know existed. This love is the most unconditional, completely consuming love the human brain and heart are capable of feeling. Sometimes it is difficult to understand that Jesus loves us even more than we love our children. Again, God had put someone in my path to ease my fear as we discussed the many joys of motherhood.

I told the technician I was wearing a wig and had brought a toboggan to wear during the scan. For those with little or no hair I suggest bringing some kind of toboggan-type hat to wear during the scan. It can get very cold inside the machine with your head exposed for 30 minutes. Once changed, I lay inside the machine for my second bone scan.

December 16, 2014 I just read my notes from the first bone scan. I'm trying really hard to stop the tears. We'll be leaving shortly heading to the hospital. I'll get the injection wait three hours and return for the bone scan. I am scared. I am overwhelmed. I have peace from God. Contradicting statements but all true.

As the machine slowly moved across my body, I focused on the scripture Jesus gave me only hours earlier. The evening before the scan I had been in full battle with the "what if" monster, but as hard as I fought, the "what ifs" fought harder. I picked up my Bible to aimlessly thumb through the pages. As the passages quickly passed, I glimpsed the word "bones" in one of the chapters. "Your body will glow with health, your very bones will vibrate with life!" (Proverbs 3:8 Message). I couldn't believe it, the night before my bone scan Jesus showed me this verse. He again supplied encouragement when I needed it the most. As fearful as any of the imaging tests can be, this is also an opportunity to fully rely on God. If you are battling your own "what if" beast, ask for the encouragement you need. These tough times are when we are most willing to listen for God's voice.

Peace in these situations can only come from God, and without my faith that Jesus never forsakes, I'm not sure I could have continued to lie there waiting as the machine scanned my body. Thankfully, God's spirit never left me. I am also very grateful to God for giving me technicians who so graciously helped me during both scans.

"I've believed as many as six impossible things before breakfast."
Lewis Carroll, Alice's Adventures in Wonderland

CHAPTER 23

Things People Do and Say (or Shouldn't Do and Say)

All of the following I have either experienced or someone has shared their experience with me. I know no one has malicious intent but words can be encouraging or stir fear. We all need to choose our words carefully, especially when talking with someone who has a life altering diagnosis.

DO use positive words when discussing the future. We all know cancer is unpredictable but it can also be curable or manageable. There is enough negative information; we need words of hope and encouragement.

DO think of the implications of your words. Once, as I offered condolences to a woman whose sister had recently passed away, she said, "I wish I were talking with my sister rather than you." The statement caught me so off guard I asked her to repeat it . . . twice! She repeated it both times without hesitation. Later, when Dan and I discussed the conversation, we agreed she probably meant she wished we were both alive. At least that's what I choose to believe.

DO volunteer help. I was truly blessed with supportive family and loving friends who helped take care of Alana and me through my diagnosis and treatments. One of the biggest gestures you can offer is to help their kids maintain some form of normalcy. Offer to take them to the playground, movies, dinner, etc. Bringing dinner is always helpful but if that's not your strength, take a gift card. Chick-fil-A is perfect for those with kids; it's a great meal for all ages. Panera gift cards were also much-appreciated during my treatments. Try to choose a restaurant that offers a variety of foods.

Do use humor when appropriate. Laughter is good medicine. Use it whenever possible but never at someone's expense. If you look long and hard you can almost always see something humorous within any difficult situation.

When someone is diagnosed with cancer DON'T emphasize to anyone that they waited before going to the doctor. Though it may not be intended this way, that attitude implies blame. Saying a woman should have gone to the doctor earlier could imply she could have done something to prevent the situation.

DON'T ask detailed questions about someone's surgery/reconstruction unless they volunteer the information. We all have a curious tendency to want to know all the gory details but unless someone willingly offers this information, don't ask. Please do not inquire if they had reconstruction or not, did they have nipple-sparing surgery (yes, someone actually asked that question), did they have a single mastectomy or a double, will they have more reconstruction, this list could go on endlessly.

DON'T call someone a cancer patient. When these words are spoken we visualize a very sick person shriveled up in a bed. That's not what we look like.

DON'T hug a woman after surgery. I know you have the best intentions but you have no idea what's going on in her chest area. Whether she's had a mastectomy, lumpectomy, or reconstruction, it hurts. Nerves are reconnecting, the surrounding tissue is sore, and everything is trying to heal. Just pat her on the back or, if you must hug, make it a gentle side hug.

DON'T classify cancer into "good" and "bad" categories. While sitting in the chemo chair getting treatment, I heard two other women talking about the "bad" breast cancer. Both of these women were told by their physicians they had the "best possible scenario." Turns out I had the "bad" type no one wanted. I didn't realize there was a type anyone wanted. Be careful what you say. You don't know who is listening or what the other person may have been through or may be facing.

DON'T use qualifying words when talking about recurrence. April 2014 someone asked me, "Has your cancer come back yet?" Yes, that was the question. "Yet" implies inevitability. Though I understand no harm was intended, the question was appalling. I strongly suggest to all those reading, choose your words carefully. Do not imply the cancer will return or infer any other prediction.

DON'T stare at someone's chest. My friends have deemed this the three-second rule, but I think it should be limited to two. After a breast cancer diagnosis, people look at your chest. The second we look away people want to steal a two-second (my friends think three) glance. Just know, we know what you're doing. We notice those glances and sideways stares.

DON'T touch. There comes a point when people stop gawking over your chest and become more concerned with your hair (or lack thereof). Whatever your situation—wig, scarf, hat, bald head—people want to touch your head. It's like the pregnant lady whose belly is constantly being touched by strangers. Don't touch the hair. First of all, our immune system is compromised and we're trying to avoid unnecessary contact. Secondly (and maybe more importantly), if we are wearing a wig we're already paranoid it will move, touching it only increases the chances.

DON'T describe the future as uncertain. I once talked with a woman who was many years past her diagnosis. As we spoke of our worries, she told me she understood the fear of our future being uncertain. As with most statements, I knew she didn't have ill intent. However, hearing that my future could be uncertain, or that I might not have a future, pierced through my heart.

DON'T relay statistical information unless requested. Hearing negative statistics can be devastating. We're all grateful for medical advancements, but sometimes we just can't bear to hear another statistic. Someone in the medical profession once told me, "If you had come in with this same diagnosis a few years earlier, you would have been written off." I know she was trying to emphasize how far medical treatments have come, but knowing my diagnosis had once been viewed as a death sentence was not something I wanted to hear.

Don't refer to anyone as a "goner" (yep, heard that one too). I'm sure it was well-intentioned, but I heard a lady tell another who was in treatment that if she were in another country she would have been a "goner."

- PART V -

Regaining Normalcy

(or so I thought)

"What you do for yourself dies with you. What you do for others and the world remains and is immortal."
Albert Pine

CHAPTER 24

You Won't Believe What Happened Next

On March 14, 2013, a couple of weeks after we returned from Disney, I had a hysterectomy. There were no complications and no additional cancer was found. My oncology gynecologist and I had discussed the hysterectomy, and I understood I would have four new incisions on my abdomen and one incision "down there" (yes, that's the medical terminology here in the South). I felt peace going into the surgery, truly believing there was no cancer in my body.

I went home the day after surgery, March 15, with minimal recovery time. If you are given the choice, consider staying the one night offered. Why not let well-experienced nurses take charge of your care all while other people make and bring you food. It was a good combination.

Recovery from the hysterectomy was surprisingly easy. There were days I was tired or slightly sore but certainly not painful or unmanageable. When I went for a follow-up appointment, my surgeon said all was healing as expected. Shortly afterward, my family and I went to the Smoky Mountains; life was good and incredibly normal. I was relieved, assuming the hysterectomy would be my last surgery. Boy, was I in for a surprise! I had no idea what lay ahead.

*****

The weekend of June 25, 2013, Dan and I left for an overnight trip to a (somewhat) nearby State Park. We planned to hike (my favorite), canoe, and eat (both our favorites). Once there, we walked to the boat dock to decide between renting a canoe or paddle boat. As we stood there surrounded by God's beautiful creation, I felt an odd sensation, almost as if I had involuntarily urinated. I went to the restroom and realized something was in fact coming out of my body, but it wasn't urine. There was a small amount of blood and other fluids. I was shocked when I realized there was also a mass of what appeared to be an organ pushing its way out of my body. I attempted to push whatever it was back, but the pain was tremendous and getting worse. Bent over, I managed to walk the short distance back to Dan.

I could barely speak but I told him I needed to go to the emergency room. I can only imagine his shock. One minute we're discussing canoeing and the next I'm in tremendous pain asking to go to the nearest hospital. Dan was so frightened he practically carried me to the car, then drove to the ranger's station and called an ambulance. I lay in the car as he held my hand waiting for the ambulance.

The EMT who rode in the back was sympathetic as he took my blood pressure and pulse. It was obvious he was alarmed by the results but assured me we would arrive at the hospital soon. He repeatedly told me, "You stay with me." I assumed he meant either stay conscience or alive. The EMT had no idea how determined I was to "stay with him." He didn't know what I had been through or the magnitude of my will to live. I understood the power of the brain and focused completely on staying conscience. Among the chaos, I knew the Holy Spirit was with me.

Once we arrived at the hospital, I lay there holding this mass of what I now assumed to be my bladder. When I felt it starting to protrude, I would push the organ back inside my body until I could no longer bear the pain. I had heard of people needing bladder repair but I knew mine was completely intact before the hysterectomy. I had no other ideas as to what else could be happening. At this point I was attempting to convince myself I would need a bladder tack and would return to Chattanooga for the surgery.

My attempts at self-diagnosing weren't working; I allowed the fear of not knowing to consume me. I quickly realized something worse was happening and there was a chance I might not survive. I thought death could be a real and immediate possibility. Whatever this was, it continued to slowly come out of my body. I thought of my precious daughter. I began to desperately tell Dan to consistently encourage Alana's walk with God and always remind her how much I love her. I went on with my pleas while he tried to reassure me I was going to be okay. I still don't know if he actually believed what he spoke, but I wanted to believe. I pleaded with God to spare my life.

The emergency room doctor ordered a CT scan of my abdomen. When they rolled my bed into the scan room, I felt almost as if I was in the twilight zone. It all seemed surreal. How did I go from planning a hike to waiting for a CT scan in the ER? "What if they found additional cancer?" "What if something was terribly wrong and they needed to do emergency surgery?" "What if I couldn't make it back to Chattanooga?" I had told Dan I did not want to have an operation at that hospital. I emphatically asked to be taken back to Chattanooga but I also realized there was a possibility I wouldn't be able to travel. During the scan the technician told Dan he could stay and watch as my scan came through his computer. The technician explained he saw something in my lower abdomen and believed my bladder was very low. I would later learn he was wrong.

I was moved back to triage while the radiologist read the scan. One of the nurses, who knew of my cancer diagnosis, told me she had overheard the doctor saying the scan didn't show anything suspicious of cancer. This was an enormous relief. After requesting numerous times, the ER doctor came in to do a gynecological exam. This was the first time I had ever wanted one! The nurse told me the bed was not equipped for the exam, meaning it didn't have those lovely stirrups us females must hoist our feet into. To accommodate, the nurse discretely slid an upside-down bed pan under me. To make matters worse, they had to rotate my bed facing the wall because the curtain (yes curtain, not door) wouldn't completely close. Anyone walking past could witness my exam and supposed extruding bladder. The ER doctor appeared nervous and uncertain. After the exam he hesitantly said he thought the protruding mass was my bladder. His puzzled expression told me he was not the least bit confident with the diagnosis. Although my confidence in anything going on around me was gone, I wanted to believe him but deep in my heart I felt he was wrong. He told us to go back to the cabin, rest, and return to Chattanooga as soon as possible in the morning.

Dan and I discussed going back to Chattanooga but agreed we should follow the doctor's instructions and return the following morning. It was late by the time we settled in at the cabin. I had successfully pushed most of whatever was protruding back inside my body. Throughout most of the night, I laid on my back awake. Nothing out of the ordinary happened but the following morning, once I stood to go to the bathroom, the mass started to come through. It was painful as I pushed it back into my body but not unbearable. Dan begged me to let him call an ambulance to get me back to Chattanooga but I insisted that wasn't necessary. In hindsight, I should have conceded. But I still believed this mass was my bladder and that it could be fixed once we returned. Dan helped me to the car and we began the drive.

Not long after we were on the road, I called my gynecologist's office. The nurse quickly returned my call and, after I briefly explained the recent events, she said, "I don't want to alarm or scare you but the mass may not be your bladder." She asked how much longer before we were back in Chattanooga. She was so kind and compassionate as she told me the mass was most likely my intestines, not my bladder. She assured me the surgeon would be there waiting once we arrived. I can't remember exactly what she said but she wished I were in an ambulance. I now agreed with my nurse and Dan that I should be in an ambulance.

When we arrived, the nurse met us in the parking lot with a wheelchair. As promised, the doctor was waiting, literally standing in the hallway. He completed only a brief exam before stating the mass was definitely not my bladder. My small intestines were coming out of my body. He asked if the attending physician did an exam. He shook his head in disbelief when I told him of the CT scan and the protruding bladder diagnosis. Even if that diagnosis had been correct, they were astounded that medical professionals would release me with instructions to return to a cabin overnight and then ride two hours with an extruding organ.

My surgeon explained he was going to push as much of the organs back into my body as possible. He said to stop him when the pain became unbearable and they would take me to surgery. I cried as he pushed. Dan was sitting beside my exam table with his head down. He was clearly upset. My husband had to sit helplessly as the surgeon continued to push organs back inside my body. Once I could no longer tolerate the pain I asked the doctor to stop. I was then admitted to the hospital and prepped for organ reconstruction surgery.

My mom and dad met us at the hospital and stayed by my side just as they had since the beginning of my journey. I vividly remember their look of despair and fear as I was wheeled to the operating room. I can only imagine the shock they felt as Dan explained the situation. My mom and dad had been through everything with me since the initial diagnosis. Their strength, courage, and complete belief that God would again spare my life helped me more than they will ever know.

I don't remember much about the operating room, but there were several nurses and techs surrounding my bed. My last memory before going to sleep was the tech asking if I could help move my body from the bed to the operating table. I remember trying to help but that's the last memory.

June 26, 2013, exactly one year from the hematoma surgery, I had complete vaginal cuff repair and organ reconstruction surgery. Around three in the morning one of the physicians who had assisted during surgery came to check on me. He asked what I remembered immediately before surgery. I recalled the information I could, and then he began to describe what took place after I was asleep. He said once they moved me to the end of the operating table and lifted my legs, my intestines fell out of my body. According to the physician, my intestines "hit the floor and the nurses swooped down to get them." Yes, those were his exact words. Dan and I listened in shock, trying to grasp the reality of what had happened. I do not believe either of us could fully comprehend the magnitude of his words.

The doctor expressed his shock that I survived. He said he did not understand how we could drive almost two hours with part of my intestines protruding from my body. He was amazed they did not develop a kink or tear during my attempts to push them back or from being exposed for such a long period of time. The odds of my survival had been stacked against me. He told us if any of these or other circumstances had gone wrong, I would not have survived. As he spoke of his astonishment I said, "It was God. God was with me."

According to the doctor, I should not have made it through alive. Not only am I alive, I am healthy, my intestines are intact, and I eventually returned to all normal activities. If you ever doubt God still performs healing, these events remind us our God is a God fully capable of modern day miracles.

Friday morning, three days after surgery, I planned to be released from the hospital and go immediately to Alana's first theater performance. Dan had brought the clothes I would need to go from the hospital to Alana's school. She had been rehearsing daily for two weeks and I was determined to be there to watch the performance. Unfortunately my body did not cooperate. Because part of my intestines had been outside my body, I was given strong antibiotics to fight the possibility of infection. During the second night following surgery I became violently ill. Throughout the night, Dan and the nurse rotated bringing me containers. The nausea and vomiting continued until morning. It was a rough night, not only for me but I know the night was long for both Dan and my nurse. When the doctor came in that morning, I told him of my plan to be dismissed. Understandably, his plan did not agree with mine. I needed to remain in the hospital until they were certain an infection wasn't forming.

My heart ached as Dan left to join our family. Thankfully, my precious dad came to stay with me despite my attempts to assure him I would be fine alone. We talked quietly as I watched the clock knowing the play would soon begin. As I sat in bed fighting back the tears, God again used a negative experience to teach me an important lesson. He reminded me that in the big picture of life this was only one event. Alana would have many future adventures and I planned to be there for as many as possible.

It wasn't long before Alana and my family came to tell me all about the play. She beamed with pride as she described the details and how much fun she had. I was sad when she and my sister-in-law left the hospital but thanked God again for the people who love Alana and helped her life continue as close to normal as possible. I stayed in the hospital four days then returned home with antibiotics and a heart filled with gratitude to be alive.

"I will not die but live, and will proclaim what the Lord has done."
Psalm 118:17 (NIV)

CHAPTER 25

Whatever Normal Means

I wrote down the events of my intestinal reconstruction on July 3, 2013, a couple of weeks after the event. During the weeks between I was conflicted, questioning why I was alive and why God had granted me life over and over again. The following is taken directly from my record of daily events as I wrestled with the purpose behind the complications:

I stopped writing shortly after this event. I returned home and continued to recover but each day felt almost as if I were living in a fog. Some might describe it as a depressive state, but I didn't feel depressed. I was filled with gratitude but also struggling as I questioned the purpose behind the recent events. Have you ever wondered if something was a miracle? Was it luck? Was it bad luck? Was it coincidence? Was life on auto pilot or was the Holy Spirit guiding each step? The unanswered speculations continued during the weeks and months of recovery.

As grateful as I was, it took a while to emotionally recover. Adjusting

July 2013 2 Corinthians 5:15 tells us "And He died for all, that those who live should live no longer for themselves but for Him who died for them and rose again." Our lives are not ours to live here on this earth, but our lives are to be lived to honor God. I do not know why God has spared me from the diagnosis and later from complications that could have quickly taken my life. Although I do not understand why, I am indescribably grateful. I want to tell everyone what He has done and that, regardless of the situation, He will never leave us.

to the thought of "I could have died but didn't" is a process. Though I had been confronted with death in the past, this was different. This accident was an acute, emergency situation that came quickly and without warning. After most of us go through trauma, we live in a surreal state trying to process the knowledge of potential death. And it takes time. Our bodies recover but sometimes our brain must play catch-up. In the time following the intestinal reconstruction, I experienced an intense emotional journey. Though I was filled with overwhelming gratitude for simply being alive, I truly didn't understand the purpose. There were times during this emotional mending when I questioned why it all happened. Was I supposed to write about these experiences? What does God want me do with these life events? Should I do nothing? Should I wait? The questions swirled inside my head.

A turning point began during a night spent with friends. One of my closet friends came with her children to cook dinner at my house. As we sat around the table laughing and sharing stories, something clicked. I couldn't continue to be afraid of the "what if." The past year had brought complications and unexpected surgeries but I did not want to live in fear of what the future might hold. God had granted life today, this very moment. When we find ourselves emotionally cowering in fear of when health could again be snatched away, we must ask Jesus to give us the strength and courage to focus only on the gratitude of the moment and take the fear of the unknown from us.

Two years after I was diagnosed with triple negative breast cancer I had my chemo port taken out. Removing this physical link to past surgeries and treatment felt, oddly enough, sad. God had given me opportunities to meet people who were newly diagnosed and the port was my cancer veteran badge. With time I realized I didn't miss the device but missed meeting people who were just beginning their treatment journey. Most of all, I worried with the obvious physical evidence of cancer gone, would I continue to meet people within the cancer community? Would I have opportunities to encourage those going through treatment? Would I forget what God did? Would I fizzle out and live life as if it never happened? With His leadership I've told my story and experiences to others facing this journey. And now I'm telling my story to you. All in hopes that you find encouragement and a sense of normalcy from someone who's been there, even if I don't have that circular symbol still protruding from my chest.

*****

The further you go into the cancer terrain you may have friends who have a different outcome. Somewhere along this journey most of us will struggle with the question, "Why do bad things happen to good people?" Losing someone to a diagnosis you share is devastating and can bring with it an unexpected flood of both grief and gratitude. May 2013 was my first (but unfortunately not last) experience with this overwhelming combination of emotions. A few days before Mother's Day, my friend went to live eternally with Jesus. The week before we had made plans for our next get together. When I learned of her passing, I was distraught. I grieved for her, her children, and all their family. I also, selfishly, grieved for myself. My friend had been diagnosed with triple negative several months before my diagnosis. Her passing brought grief, gratitude, guilt, and a flood of fears. I was so very grateful to be alive but questioned, "Why did my friend have to die when she fought so hard to live?" "Will I die?" "Why am I alive and she's not?" I truly did not understand why this happened.

The following week an acquaintance friend passed. In an attempt to help me avoid comparing my circumstances to this precious lady's situation, someone said to me, "She waited to go to a doctor." I understand this was an innocent comment but implying someone waited once they knew there was a problem implies blame. I've heard comments such as "they waited" or "they should have gone earlier" or "they shouldn't have taken so long to have it checked." Most of us think we know what we would do but until it is felt personally, no one can understand the fear caused by even the possibility of hearing, "You have cancer." Until we are in a position of paralyzing fear, there is no way to predict how we will react. James (chapter 3) warns us regarding taming the tongue. We should all choose our words carefully, especially when stating what we would do or what someone else should have done.

If you lose someone you love for any reason it will be devastating. We must remember in all circumstances, including grief, He will never leave us. He tells us do not be afraid, do not worry but cast all our cares to Him. Over the course of this journey I have found release from fear in God's word and prayer. Philippians 4:6 says not to be anxious over anything but to make those fears known to God. The next verse tells us what will happen when we cast our worries on God: "And the peace of God, which transcends all understanding, will guard your hearts and your minds in Christ Jesus" (Philippians 4:7 NIV).

*****

June 2016, God again reminded me of His presence. But to understand the gift you must know the background: I have several plants on my deck including one hibiscus. Each winter I bring the plant inside and hope it will make it through the cold months. This past winter Dan had suggested we let the plant go and get another in the spring. He was right, it wasn't as healthy as the others and it took up a lot of space. I agreed and soon it began to fade. Each time I watered the other plants I felt sad seeing the plant withering. I have no idea why I thought it would be OK to let the plant die or why it bothered me so much when it began to wilt, but I soon realized I deeply regretted that decision. I began to frantically care for the hibiscus, each day making sure it had plenty of sunshine and water but I wasn't sure it could survive. Once spring arrived we moved it back to the deck in the best possible location. It had regained only a few tiny leaves but not a single bloom.

June 21 2016, exactly four years from the first surgery, I woke early that morning and walked outside. Much to my surprise the hibiscus had a large, incredibly beautiful bloom. The plant that had all but ceased to exist was now regaining life. As I stared at the new flower that arrived on the fourth anniversary marking the beginning of this cancer journey, I felt Jesus' presence almost as if He were standing beside me. The past four years had brought devastation, fear, pain, and illness but greater joy, contentment, and gratitude than ever before. God did not take my life but He did redirect it. The spiritual reawakening cancer brought was nothing short of a gift.

As I bring this book to a close I think of the words our pastor recently spoke. He said our lives are filled with endings and beginnings. When one journey ends another begins. As I pondered those words I was reminded there is another journey ahead.We must never forget God has granted us life for this moment and that He has a purpose for our lives. I thought of Psalm 118:17, a verse I "accidentally" came across when in a place of complete fear: "I will not die but live, and will proclaim what the Lord has done" (NIV). I say "accidentally" because I know it wasn't coincidence. I was drawn to this verse as reassurance that there was purpose in having triple negative breast cancer. Speaking openly about my faith in God didn't come naturally, and it continues to be something I work toward daily. I've heard people say they are grateful for cancer. I can't honestly say I am grateful for the cancer but I am so very grateful for the many positive experiences that came with the diagnosis. I have never felt closer to God than I did in the midst of the fear and uncertainty of my future. I'm grateful to have the opportunity to share my journey with you and for the countless times He granted safety and life. The literature regarding triple negative can be frightening and discouraging, but our God doesn't follow the literature. James (4:14) reminds us no one knows what tomorrow will bring, but we must thank God for each minute granted and know He has a purpose for all things as we encourage each other through this cancer journey.

To come back and relive your story requires revisiting each emotion; all the negatives and positives of learning you have cancer. There is a balance found during this time that enables us to look at our experience from an objective, yet still connected stance. I said at the beginning of this book that more important than the suffering was the healing. Since recovering from all the surgeries and treatments, I'm back to normal, whatever normal means. I continue follow-ups with both my surgeon and oncologist. I have more activities jammed into my routine than anyone should ever attempt. My life is filled with all the daily activities of living that I enjoy more than the English language can describe. Alana is now in middle school and is the light of my world. Her constant love, laughter, and reassurance continue to be my greatest source of inspiration. Dan continues to make me laugh, sometimes even at myself. His devotion to me and our family has never wavered. My parents have been beside me every step of this journey. They continue to be my greatest fans and supporters; words cannot express how proud I am to be their daughter. I am alive and life continues. I've always had a great life. Now I have an even more grateful life.

WEBSITE:
SharonRatchford.com

EMAIL:
Sharon@SharonRatchford.com

FACEBOOK:
Facebook.com/SharonRatchfordBook

BLOG:
SharonRatchford.Wordpress.com

"When you have exhausted all possibilities, remember this: you haven't."
Thomas Edison

BREAST CANCER
SUPPORT RESOURCES

When in the midst of a cancer diagnosis, you will receive a lot of information from your medical team, family, and friends. While the influx of information is generous, it can feel as if you're drinking from a fire hose. Focus on what you need in the moment, allowing yourself time to learn what will be needed in the future. The list below gives breast cancer support resources from research sites, appearance-related services, support groups, and family services. Remember, some of these will help you immediately and others you won't need until you're further along with recovery.

BREAST CANCER RESEARCH

Breastcancer.org *(breastcancer.org)* – This non-profit organization offers updated and reliable information about breast cancer.

American Institutes for Cancer Research *(aicr.org)* – American Institutes for Cancer Research focuses on the practical application of nutrition links to cancer and your daily diet.

Cancer Treatment Centers of America *(cancercenter.com)* – This network of fully-accredited cancer hospitals focuses on treating patients in all aspects of their journey with cancer from diagnosis through treatment. Locations are listed on their website.

National Cancer Institute *(cancer.gov)* – NCI is the primary government agency dedicated to cancer research and training. Coordinating with the National Cancer Program, NCI is a large contributor to cancer research and the support of cancer-related organizations across the country.

National Comprehensive Cancer Network *(nccn.org)* – NCCN is an alliance of leading cancer centers that focus on research and education as well as patient care. All hospitals follow NCCN Guidelines for patient care at all stages of treatment.

Dr. Susan Love Research Foundation *(drsusanloveresearch.org)* – Through project-based, collaborative efforts, this foundation seeks to find the gaps in breast cancer research and create solutions.

Susan G. Komen *(5.komen.org)* – The Susan G. Komen organization is an excellent place to find updated research, support services, and a plethora information about breast cancer from diagnosis to survivorship.

The University of Texas MD Anderson Cancer Center *(mdanderson.org)* – MD Anderson is a leading medical center solely dedicated to treating and educating cancer patients as well as performing research for cancer eradication and prevention. Though located in Houston, Texas, MD Anderson also has other locations across the US. Visit their website for links to information and center locations.

Vanderbilt-Ingram Cancer Center *(vicc.org)* – VICC is one of 47 institutes across the US focused on a patient-centered approach to cancer research, prevention, and treatment. You can schedule an appointment at the Nashville, Tennessee, location through their website.

Sarah Cannon Cancer Resource Center *(sarahcannon.com)* – The oncology arm of Hospital Corporation of America (HCA), Sarah Cannon offers cutting edge, advanced therapies to those facing a cancer diagnosis. Spread throughout the US and UK, you can find the center closest to you on their website.

APPEARANCE RESOURCES

Look Good Feel Better *(lookgoodfeelbetter.org)* – On a mission to improve the self-esteem of women undergoing cancer treatment, this organization offers complimentary beauty sessions to aid women in combating appearance-based side effects. Local, statewide, and national workshops are done by trained professionals. You can find programs near you on their website.

Good Wishes *(goodwishesscarves.org)* – This non-profit provides a free scarf or head wrap to anyone experiencing hair loss during treatment. In addition to the head covering, each woman's name and city is put on a placard on the Wall of Hope at the Good Wishes office as a way of reminding staff of those in need of positive thoughts.

Knitted Knockers *(knittedknockers.org)* – Eliminating the need for expensive and heavy traditional prosthetics, Knitted Knockers provides women who have undergone breast surgery free handmade breast prosthetics from yarn. These soft prosthetics fit inside a regular bra to give the look and feel of having breasts post-mastectomy or in the midst of reconstruction. You can request a knocker (or two) on their website, as well as donate financially or skillfully by knitting knockers for others.

SUPPORT RESOURCES

The Gracie Foundation, Inc. *(thegraciefoundationinc.org)* – Started after its founder, Gail "Gracie" Germain's, experience with breast cancer, The Gracie Foundation creates and sends free gift packages to women undergoing breast cancer treatment. This non-profit organization is headquartered in Florida and packages include items such as lip balm, scarves, soaps, and inspirational journals. You can refer those undergoing treatment and make donations through their website.

MyLifeline.org *(mylifeline.org)* – A non-profit organization, MyLifeline helps those going through cancer and their caregivers form a support community through the creation of a free, personalized website.

Cancer Community Center *(cancercommunitycenter.org)* – Located in South Portland, Maine, the Cancer Community Center offers free support services and programs to those living with cancer and their families.

Cleaning for a Reason *(cleaningforareason.org)* – Since 2006, Cleaning for a Reason has been providing free house cleaning services to women undergoing cancer treatment so they can focus on their health and not their house. Applications are available on their website.

American Cancer Society, Reach to Recovery *(cancer.org)* – Using breast cancer survivor volunteers, Reach to Recovery helps women cope with the emotional unease of breast cancer from as early as the possibility of a diagnosis. Filter for "Reach to Recovery" in the search bar of the American Cancer Society homepage to find a program near you.

CancerCare *(cancercare.org)* – Providing free support services for those diagnosed with cancer, CancerCare helps people manage the difficulties of cancer through free support groups, educational workshops, and financial assistance.

Living Beyond Breast Cancer *(lbbc.org)* – Living Beyond Breast Cancer offers programs, up-to-date information, and support to those undergoing breast cancer treatment.

FOR FAMILIES

Kids Konnected *(kidskonnected.org)* – Started by an 11-year-old boy whose mother was diagnosed with breast cancer, this California-based non-profit offers support services and resource material for children and teens who have a parent diagnosed with cancer or have lost a parent to cancer. You can also send a care package to a child in one of these two situations through their website.

FOR SURVIVORS

PearlPoint Cancer Support *(my.pearlpoint.org)* – This nonprofit charity provides information and guidance to those impacted by a cancer diagnosis. While the site offers helpful information for those diagnosed about the journey of cancer, the site also has an in-depth supportive Survivorship Handbook that is an excellent resource for those out of treatment.

Breast Cancer Support Services *(bcss-chattanooga.org)* – BCSS is a non-profit organization in Chattanooga that caters to those undergoing breast cancer treatment as well as survivors. With a board of directors made up of local medical professionals and volunteers, BCSS offers many free programs, including:

- *Emergency Fund* – financial assistance for qualifying low-income families during breast cancer treatment
- *Support Groups* – professionally facilitated peer groups for female breast cancer survivors at any length of survivorship
- *On With Life, Therapy Group* – professionally facilitated group for women with metastatic breast cancer
- *Mastectomy Bra and Prosthesis Bank* – provided for free to women in need and at any length of survivorship
- *Wig Referral Service* – collaboration with professional stylists who provide wigs for those undergoing chemo
- *Educational Series* – quarterly educational programs with area medical and health professionals regarding breast cancer
- *Moving On* – annual health and fitness workshop designed to provide breast cancer survivors with information, tips, and a variety of workouts to live a healthy life post-cancer

Wig Palace *(thewigpalace.com)* – This is where I found my wigs while going through chemotherapy. The Wig Palace is a wonderful resource for wigs, extensions, scarves, hats, and many other head coverings and accessories.

Rees Skillern Cancer Institute *(memorial.org/cancer-institute)* – Located at CHI Memorial Hospital, Rees Skillern is the leading provider in Chattanooga for cancer-related services. There are seven centers of excellence as part of the institute, including the MaryEllen Locher Breast Center of Excellence. This institute offers up-to-date treatment technology in radiation therapy for those with certain types of cancer. Also part of the Rees Skillern is the Joe and Virginia Schmissrauter Centers for Cancer Support, where those diagnosed and their families can receive support services such as peer groups and educational material.

MaryEllen Locher Breast Center of Excellence *(memorial.org/maryellen-locher-breast-center)* – This all-inclusive center of excellence offers quality, time-efficient breast care to women in the city of Chattanooga and surrounding areas. Established in 2007, The MaryEllen Locher Breast Center can offer a full range of services, such as moving from a screening mammogram to diagnostic work, all in one appointment to help alleviate the concern and hassle of scheduling multiple appointments. This breast center is part of CHI Memorial Hospital's Rees Skillern Cancer Institute.

Erlanger Cancer Resource Center *(Erlanger.org)* – Erlanger Health Systems in Chattanooga offers a variety of cancer resources for those facing a diagnosis.

Erlanger is the first and only regional cancer center to use CyberKnife in treatment, a robotic piece of radiation technology that treats tumors. They also have a board of certified genetic counselors for those seeking genetic testing, as well as other resources. Visit the Erlanger website and search for "Cancer/Oncology" under the "Medical Services" tab.

Pink Petal Boutique *(accessfamilypharmacy.com)* – Located inside Access Family Pharmacy in Hixson, Pink Petal Boutique is a mastectomy boutique where women can purchase breast forms, bras, and an assortment of head coverings and accessories after surgery and during treatment. As part of this locally-owned pharmacy that's been a part of the Chattanooga community for over 60 years, the boutique offers a comfortable and private place for women going through breast cancer to try on and purchase appearance-related items they may need during their diagnosis.

American Cancer Society, Chattanooga location *(cancer.org)* – The American Cancer Society has a local office in Chattanooga, as well as an office in most major cities. You can visit their local office to get relevant information regarding your diagnosis. To find office hours, address, and phone numbers, go to the American Cancer Society website and click the "Find Local ACS" tab. Filter using your zip code for more information.

Sarah Cannon Center, Chattanooga location *(parkridgemedicalcenter.com)* – Located at Parkridge Medical Center, the Chattanooga Sarah Cannon Cancer Center provides a plethora of diagnostic and treatment services for breast cancer. As part of their state-of-the-art treatment options, this is the only location in Chattanooga that offers Intraoperative Radiation Therapy (IORT), a special type of radiation therapy that is delivered in its entirety at the time of surgery. This service is given to those undergoing a lumpectomy with negative lymph nodes that meet certain qualifying criteria. Though still considered a clinical trial, the results of this new technology have shown to be very effective in treatment.

GLOSSARY OF TERMS
& DEFINITIONS*

A/C treatment – A combination of chemotherapy drugs used to treat breast cancer. Combines Doxorubicin (AKA Adriamycin) and Cyclophosphamide (AKA Cytoxan).

Adjuvant chemotherapy – Chemotherapy that is given to patients after they have had surgery to remove all visible cancer. The follow-up chemo is used to kill any unseen cancer cells that may have been left behind so new tumors don't grow and the cells don't spread.

B.A.R.T (genetic testing) – A genetic test that looks for certain genes the BRCA test does not. This test is usually recommended to only those with a strong family history of breast cancer because it can be expensive.

Benign – Non-cancerous.

Biopsy – A procedure that takes tissue samples from a mass, which are then tested to determine if cancer is present.

BRCA gene test – A blood test that analyzes a patient's DNA to determine whether they carry one of two breast cancer genes, BRCA1 and BRCA2.

Contained cancer – When the cancer stays within the breast and doesn't spread. This is stages 0-3.

Diagnosis – The identification of an illness.

Drains – Drainage tubes are surgically inserted in the chest to relieve pressure on the lungs and remove fluid from the area. The tube is inserted through the skin and muscles between the ribs and into the chest cavity.

Ductal Carcinoma in situ (DCIS) – Non-invasive, "in place" cancer. The abnormal cells are located in the milk ducts of the breast and have not spread outward to the breast tissue. DCIS can also be called "pre-invasive" or "pre-cancerous" because there is a possibility of the abnormal cells spreading.

Estrogen receptor type cancer – One of three receptor types of breast cancer. If a cancer is classified as ER-positive, then the cancer cells contain a receptor that produces and attaches to estrogen (a female hormone).

Echocardiogram – A test that monitors heart activity.

Fluid pocket – Body fluids can build up in a place where tissue has been removed by surgery. Fluid pockets can occur after such procedures as a lumpectomy, mastectomy, or lymph node removal.

Grades of cancer – The classification of abnormal cells in comparison to normal cells. There are three grades a mass can be categorized as, ranging from slow growing to quick growing. See chapter 7 for a full break down.

Hematoma – A blood clot.

HER2 – Human Epidermal Growth Factor Receptor 2 is one of three receptor types of breast cancer. If a cancer is classified as HER2-positive, then the cancer cells contain a receptor that produces and attaches to this protein, which is involved in cell growth and survival.

Hormonal therapy – A type of treatment that blocks hormones aiding in the growth of cancer cells in order to kill them. This type of treatment can be used for hormone receptor type breast cancer such as ER-positive and PR-positive.

Hysterectomy – A surgical procedure to remove the uterus and, in some cases, other female organs. This is sometimes done as a preventative measure for certain types of breast cancer.

Intravenous chemo – When chemotherapy drugs are administered directly into the bloodstream through an IV inserted in the arm.

Invasive breast cancer – The abnormal cells (cancer) spread from the original site (in the milk ducts) and into the breast tissue, possibly even the surrounding lymph nodes.

Ki-67 – In order to estimate how quickly cells are dividing into new cells, a Ki-67 test is given. Ki-67 is a cell protein that increases when cells start to divide. The test consists of a staining process that tracks the percentage of cells positive for Ki-67. The higher the percentage, the quicker they're dividing.

Lobules – Glands that produce breast milk.

Lumpectomy – Surgery to remove the tumor in the breast as well as lymph nodes surrounding the breast. The rest of the breast is left intact. Lumpectomy procedures are usually followed by radiation treatment.

Lymphedema – The collection of lymph, a waste removing fluid, in one area of the body that causes the area to swell. This can occur after breast cancer surgery or radiation because nodes or vessels through which lymph once travelled could be damaged, prohibiting the fluid to move through the tissue as it once did.

Lymph nodes – Small organs that fight infection and can be found in the breast (internal mammary), under the arms (axillary), in the neck (cervical), and above the collarbone (supraclavicular).

Malignant – Cancerous.

Mastectomy – Surgery to remove the cancerous tumor, which involves removing the entire breast. The types of mastectomy are: partial (removes more than a lumpectomy but not the whole breast), single (removes the entire breast that contains the mass), and bi-lateral (removes both breasts).

Metastatic cancer – This is cancer that has spread beyond the breast and into other organs, such as the lungs, liver, bones, or brain. This is also known as stage 4 or advanced breast cancer.

Neoadjuvant chemotherapy – Chemo treatment that is done before surgery. Though this doesn't affect the likelihood of a recurrence, neoadjuvant treatment does allow for doctors to see how the tumor responds to drugs, as well as shrinks the size of the tumor to make surgery less extensive.

Neulasta – A drug that is given after some chemotherapy treatments to boost white blood cells.

Non-invasive breast cancer – The abnormal cells (cancer) have not left the original site and are still in the milk ducts.

Nurse navigator – A medical professional who will help those in the midst of a cancer diagnosis navigate through the medical community. A nurse navigator can help alleviate the burden of the logistics of treatment while you focus on getting better.

Oncologist – A doctor who specializes in and treats cancer. This is usually the person who manages the patient's care and treatment after diagnosis.

Paclitaxel treatment – A type of drug used in chemotherapy treatment.

Pathology – The study of disease cause and effect, particularly laboratory examination of body tissue for medical diagnosis or forensic purposes.

Port – A port is used in a type of chemotherapy. Inserted during outpatient surgery, a port is a quarter-sized disc that is placed directly under the skin. A catheter connects the port to a large vein in the chest and chemo medicines are given through a special needle that fits in the port. The port is removed via another outpatient surgery once chemotherapy is completed.

Progesterone cancer – One of three receptor types of breast cancer. If a cancer is classified as PR-positive, then the cancer cells contain a receptor that produces and attaches to progesterone (a female hormone).

Prognosis – The estimated course a disease will take.

Prophylactic mastectomy – Preventative surgery to remove one or both breasts. This is usually done after genetic testing to reduce the risk of developing breast cancer.

Prophylactic Oophorectomy – Preventative surgery to remove the ovaries. This is usually done after genetic testing to reduce the risk of developing ovarian cancer.

Radiation therapy – A type of cancer treatment that uses high-energy x-rays to kill cancer cells.

Reconstruction – A procedure to rebuild the breast(s) after a mastectomy. This can be done in conjunction with a mastectomy or later on down the road after treatment.

Reconstruction specialist – The surgeon who will be in charge of orchestrating and performing reconstructive surgery of the breast(s).

Recurrence – Cancer that returns after treatment is complete. The three different types of recurrence are local (when it comes back in the same place as the original diagnosis), regional (when it comes back in the lymph nodes or nearby tissue), and distant (when it returns and spreads to other parts of the body).

Remission – When, after treatment, the cancer has diminished in size and symptoms of cancer have decreased or disappeared. Though cancer cells still might be present in the body, they are no longer visible.

Sentinel node – The first lymph node to collect cancer cells and move out from the tumor. This node is found through a sentinel node dye procedure.

Sentinel node dye procedure – A procedure used to determine whether the cancer cells have spread to axillary lymph nodes or not. To do this, the surgeon injects a tracer into the breast that consists of blue ink. The first node to absorb the tracer, as indicated by their blue tint, is known as the sentinel node and is removed to be examined by the pathologist.

Stages of cancer – Staging describes the extent of the cancer within your body, which is important in estimating the course of the cancer (prognosis). The earlier the stage, the better the prognosis. It is determined by the size of the tumor, the number of lymph nodes infected, and whether or not the cancer has metastasized. There are four major stages with a number of sub-stages. For a full break down of stage, see chapter 7.

Targeted therapy – A type of treatment that targets specific genes or proteins that help cancer cells grow.

Triple negative breast cancer – A diagnosis of breast cancer that is negative to all three receptor types. Because of this, TNBC tumors do not respond to receptor targeted treatments.

BreastCancer.org, American Cancer Society, and the American Society of Clinical Oncology[1, 6, & 18].

SOURCES

(in order of appearance)

Chapter 3: *Meet Your Treatment Team*
- (1) American Cancer Society. *For Women Facing Breast Cancer.* n.p.: ACS, June 2010. Print.

Chapter 4: *Questions to Ask Your Treatment Team*
- (1) American Cancer Society. *For Women Facing Breast Cancer.* n.p.: ACS, June 2010. Print.
- (2) American Cancer Society. *Chemotherapy: What It Is, How It Helps.* n.p.: ACS, Apr. 2016. Print.

Chapter 5: *Mastectomy // My Mantra – "Thank you, Jesus, for healing!"*
- (1) American Cancer Society. *For Women Facing Breast Cancer.* n.p.: ACS, June 2010. Print.

Chapter 6: *What to Expect After Surgery // The Human Octopus Phase*
- (3) "Mastectomy: What to Expect." *Breastcancer.org,* May 2013. Web.
- (4) "5 tips from my mastectomy experience." *The University of Texas MD Anderson Cancer Center,* May 2014. Web.

Chapter 7: *Understanding Your Pathology Report*
- (5) "Contents of a Pathology Report." *Susan G. Komen,* Oct. 2015. Web.
- (6) Breastcancer.org. *"Your Guide to the Breast Cancer Pathology Report."* n.p.: Breastcancer.org, 2013. Print.

Chapter 9: *Encouragement for the Chemo Bound*
- (2) American Cancer Society. *Chemotherapy: What It Is, How It Helps.* n.p.: ACS, Apr. 2016. Print.

Chapter 10: *Chemotherapy Basics*
- (2) American Cancer Society. *Chemotherapy: What It Is, How It Helps.* n.p.: ACS, Apr. 2016. Print.
- (7) Brown, Roxanne. *Chemo: Secrets to Thriving: From someone who's been there.* NorLights Press, 2011.

Chapter 15: *Nutrition During and After Treatment*
- (8) National Cancer Institute. *Eating Hints: Before, During, and After Cancer Treatment.* n.p.: National Institute of Health, Jan. 2011. Web.
- (9) Rutledge, Jack F. MD. "Fight Cancer – From Your Kitchen Table!" *inspire: Memorial's Guide to Embracing Health.* Memorial Health Care System, fall 2011, Chattanooga, pp. 12-13. Web.

Chapter 18: *The Wonderful World of Uneventful // Prognosis ... "Good"*
- (10) PearlPoint Cancer Support. *Survivorship Handbook.* n.p.: PearlPoint, 2014. Web.

Chapter 19: *Genetic Testing*
- (6) Breastcancer.org. *Your Guide to the Breast Cancer Pathology Report."* n.p.: Breastcancer.org, 2013. Print.
- (11) "Facts for Life: Genetics and Breast Cancer." *Susan G. Komen,* Sept. 2015. Web.
- (12) "BRACAnalysis Large Rearrangement Test (BART)." *Myriad Pro.* Web.

Chapter 21: *Controlling the "What If" Monster // Scripture and Cupcakes are a Powerful Combination*
- (13) National Comprehensive Cancer Network. *NCCN Guidelines for Patients: Breast Cancer Early-Stage, Stages I and II.* Fort Washington, PA: NCCN, 2016. Web.
- (14) National Comprehensive Cancer Network. *NCCN Guidelines for Patients: Stage III Breast Cancer.* Fort Washington, PA: NCCN, 2014. Web.
- (15) "Depression." *American Cancer Society,* June 2015. Web.
- (16) "Depression (PDQ) – Health Professional Version." *National Cancer Institute,* Mar. 2016. Web.
- (17) "What is Cognitive Behavior Therapy (CBT)?" *Beck Cognitive Behavior Therapy.* Web.

Glossary of Terms and Definitions
- (1) American Cancer Society. *For Women Facing Breast Cancer.* n.p.: ACS, June 2010. Print.
- (6) Breastcancer.org. *Your Guide to the Breast Cancer Pathology Report."* n.p.: Breastcancer.org, 2013. Print.
- (18) American Society of Clinical Oncology. *ASCO Answers: Breast Cancer.* n.p.: ASCO, n.d. Web.

I reference scripture a number of times throughout this book. The translations used in this book and their abbreviations are as follows:

- *Amplified Bible (AMP)*
- *English Standard Version (ESV)*
- *The Message*
- *New International Version (NIV)*
- *New King James Version (NKJV)*